A HOLISTIC GUIDE FOR EVERYDAY LIVING

Anatomy of The Human Fabric Trilogy

By Andrew R. Sadock

A comprehensive series of books designed to guide you through virtually any routine or extraordinary situation, to help you navigate any relationship, and to reveal your unique life purpose and life service through a time-proven, ancient prescription.

A HOLISTIC GUIDE FOR EVERYDAY LIVING
150 ESSENTIAL LIFE LESSONS

An easy-to-read reference book presenting practical guidance for gracefully navigating contemporary situations based upon ancient wisdom. A pragmatic adaptation of the renowned book of Chinese Taoist wisdom, the *Tao Te Ching*, complemented by other visionary, inspiring philosophies and the author's experience as a practitioner in the realm of holistic (mind-body) energy-work.

CONSCIOUS RELATIONSHIP

Using a simple analogy based upon ancient philosophy, this book answers the following questions: What is the higher purpose of relationship? Why do we attract whom we attract? What keeps a couple together in the long run? The book illuminates how various factors (natural timing, intention, communication, and the mechanisms of the subconscious mind) affect relationship.

VOICE OF THE SOUL
A CALL TO ACTION

A synopsis of personal transformation. Three types of activity innately unlock access to the wisdom of the soul—via dreams, intuitions, and synchronicity—revealing one's unique life purpose and life service.

A HOLISTIC GUIDE FOR EVERYDAY LIVING

150 Essential Life Lessons

Anatomy of the Human Fabric Trilogy, Volume One

ANDREW R. SADOCK

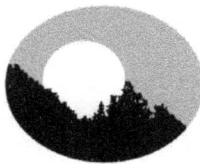

Wisdom Moon Publishing
2013

A HOLISTIC GUIDE FOR EVERYDAY LIVING
150 ESSENTIAL LIFE LESSONS

Anatomy of the Human Fabric, Volume One

Copyright © 2013 Wisdom Moon Publishing LLC

Published by Wisdom Moon Publishing LLC
San Diego, CA, USA

Wisdom Moon™, the Wisdom Moon logo™, *Wisdom Moon Publishing*™, and *WMP*™ are trademarks of Wisdom Moon Publishing LLC.

www.WisdomMoonPublishing.com

ISBN 978-1-938459-08-5 (softcover, alk. paper)
ISBN 978-1-938459-23-8 (eBook)

LCCN 2013952469

Table of Contents

Preamble

This comprehensive reference book is inspired by the renowned text of Chinese wisdom, the *Tao Te Ching* (dated as early as the late-fourth century B.C.E.), equally valid and relevant teachings from other ancient cultures (centered in Asia, Africa, Europe and the Middle East), professional experience of the author during years he served as an energyworker, and personal experience of the author.

Since long before the re-opening of China's gates to the Western world (following the Great Proletarian Cultural Revolution which transpired from 1966 to 1976), both ancient and contemporary Chinese writings regarding Eastern wisdom have been exported to the Western world. Unfortunately, at times the wisdom contained within these texts is presented using terms and concepts that are not readily understood by readers not already familiar with the subject matter.

This text presents an expansive body of timeless wisdom in an easily digestible format, with the hope that it may inspire practical application of this loving, compassionate way of being.

> *Paradox:*
> *Defies common sense*
> *and yet may be true.*
>
> Webster's Dictionary

The *Tao Te Ching* is written in the form of a paradox. A paradox is defined as a statement that defies common sense, and yet may be true. At first glance, paradoxical statements seem contrary to one another, inconsistent – and thereby untrue. Yet, deeper examination reveals a core wisdom that exposes the subtle nuances of the dualistic nature of the human condition – which serves to enhance self-awareness, our personal evolution – and cumulative evolution as a species.

> *The monkeymind abhors uncertainty.*
> *To thwart uncertainty*
> *the monkeymind takes any action necessary*
> *to attain an illusory sense of control.*

The paradox of the human condition is a direct reflection of the two divergent perspectives from which we can view any situation. We examine situations either from the perspective of the soul (soul-aligned mind), or from the perspective of the *lower* mind. The lower mind is the reactive, doubting, misinformed, unaligned fragment of the mind that craves *certainty* – i.e., abhors uncertainty. (Note that, arguably, nothing is *certain* except natural order – a.k.a. the Tao, Light, God, etc.) The lower mind is also referred to as the *monkeymind*, as it continuously squirms for certainty (again, which does not exist in the dualistic material plane). Higher mind sees only truth. It sees things as they truly are, from a compassionate and loving yet objective vantage point. The lower mind does not see truth. Rather, it *attaches* (clings) to the magnetic illusion of *homeostasis* (unchanging conditions a.k.a. certainty). The lower mind is attracted to people, objects, and events which momentarily may bring a perceived feeling of safety, but in the long-run this is nothing more than a fleeting, false sense of certainty. Everything is impermanent and so changes – except the Tao, the great eternal force and wisdom that creates, permeates, and surrounds all aspects of nature.

Certain terms, phrases, and concepts described within the *Tao Te Ching* challenge Western understanding. These terms are dissected to their essence in this book, and are then described using the simplest language to ease comprehension and application.

How to Use This Book

This text is a daily guidebook,
a daily reference to help you navigate life's
routine and extraordinary situations.
Scan the Table of Contents for a topic of interest
and turn to that page.
Ascertain the ancient wisdom
based upon the foundation of the *Tao Te Ching*
and other systems of holistic philosophy.

Please note that this book does not have to be read cover-to-cover, although it is open to that possibility. You may skim the Table of Contents for a topic of interest – an issue you currently face or simply a subject that piques your curiosity – then go to that specific discussion. Whether you choose to read the book cover-to-cover or not, some of the "A" topics, which cover some important matters, may be better understood if you give yourself the opportunity of reading them through twice, thrice or more ... and over a period of time. If you prefer reading the book cover-to-cover, consider initially taking the time to review concepts that are new to you, or, alternatively, skimming or skipping them early in your reading of this book and of this trilogy. After having a command of some more obvious and simpler-to-understand concepts, those key but more subtle ideas may make more sense when you go through them at that time, again or for the first time.

DEDICATION

This trilogy is dedicated to my brother, Jonathan Robert Sadock.
Our time together, albeit too brief, continues to inspire my path.

I miss jamming on guitar and drums after school
and playing baseball with you, Johnny!
We had a lot of fun, eh?

Your sudden absence ripped me to pieces.
Then reassembled me molecule by molecule from the inside out.
But not without help from incredible teachers — whom I never sought.
Miraculously, somehow they found me. Thank God!
They taught mostly without words and led by example.
Guess I was deemed ready for them
as I'd landed in the sub-basement of existence.

I wish no one ever had to endure such an experience.
Yet this was the defining experience of my life.
All I do, all I think, all I say
is because of you and your path.
And, in turn, the teachers
who were graciously placed before me.

You taught me much. How to love. How to let go.
But only after learning the true nature of things.
That everything is impermanent.
That all situations are perfectly designed and timed
to help us evolve.

As my greatest teacher explained using words
but only after gifting me with a 5-hour transcendent journey,
a sacred inner trek which conveyed more than words could ever say:
"It's simply a 3-D movie. It's not real ... except to the ego. [Know that] all
conditions are perfect" as they are designed to help us transcend
ego/monkeymind.

Thank you.

My dear brother, may your journey be filled with Light.

A HOLISTIC GUIDE FOR EVERYDAY LIVING
150 ESSENTIAL LIFE LESSONS

ACTION – DIRECT ACTION (DOING)

Engage in any action only after you have first achieved clarity of purpose in your mind. This assures purity of direction for the activity. If you have not yet achieved clarity of mind, first perform *non-action* to obtain clarity of mind and intention. See *Action – Non-Action.*

The path of a thousand miles begins with a single step. Then another single step. Then another single step. And so on. To accomplish a great task, engage in a series of small, direct acts. Remain focused upon each moment, each single step.

Act without expectation. Expectation alters outcome. Expectation infers focus on a future outcome. Focus in the future undermines presence of mind and thereby dilutes the power to manifest an intended outcome – and the possibility of an outcome beyond conscious expectation. Focus on the process, the task at hand, one day (i.e., one moment, one step) at a time to achieve greatest result. Future focus is a practice of ego, not soul. *The soul focuses only upon the present moment. Ego focuses in so-called past and so-called future.* The most appropriate guidance is sourced by the soul. Thus, we must focus in the present moment, exercise mindfulness, to consciously access guidance from the soul (via dreams, intuition, and synchronicity). If we expect, by definition we are focused in the so-called future. Let go of expectation (*"Let go, let God"*) to activate the possibility of manifestation far beyond expectation.

ACTION – NON-ACTION (BEING)

The term *non-action* is commonly seen throughout the *Tao Te Ching.* This term is somewhat misleading – as non-action is a form of activity (a.k.a. action), **not lack of activity.** Non-action is any activity that helps us to be present (focus upon the present moment). In energetic terms, non-action is exercise of any activity that raises our vibration. Non-action helps us *be*. Non-action IS *being*.

Being is the foundation of (right) doing.
Non-action is the foundation of right action.

Non-action varies from direct action. Again, non-action's express goal is mindfulness (focus upon the present moment). Non-action does not focus upon obtaining connection to people, objects, events, or information – i.e., material outcomes. In contrast, direct action directly intends accomplishment of a material (tangible or intangible) goal. Direct action is *doing*. Being is the foundation of right *doing*. In other words, non-action is the foundation of appropriate direct action.

For example, there are two ways to support the process of finding a new job. The obvious method is simply to peruse the classified advertisements online. Such materially-oriented activity is *direct action*. The express purpose of viewing the classified ads is to find a job. In contrast, the master (a description frequently seen in the *Tao Te Ching*) *acts without acting*. What does this mean? The master understands the connected nature of everything. S/he understands that we magnetically attract appropriate experiences (via people, objects and events) that carry/trigger appropriate lessons. By maintaining present moment focus – *through employment of non-action* (actions that support presence) – we magnetically attract the appropriate job; i.e., the job that brings appropriate lessons given our current state of evolution/awareness).

Non-action and direct action travel hand-in-hand. Non-action creates the foundation for appropriate manifestation. Non-action helps us clearly hear the voice of the soul, which guides us to appropriate experiences – experiences which bring greatest benefit at the soul level (and all subsequent levels). Without non-action, by simply taking *action*, without the clarity afforded by non-action, we may pursue opportunities that are not appropriate (e.g., *dead-end jobs* and/or other experiences that render minimal benefit at the soul or other levels). The precursor of action is non-action. In this example, non-action energetically draws us nearer to the appropriate job (which brings greatest benefit for our evolution). Non-action sends us in the right direction. Non-action subtly or not-so-subtly guides us to the knowledge of what we should do. Subsequent direct action is the action of making the telephone call or sending the email, to the appropriate employer (that we energetically attracted), and seals the deal. The ultimate benefit of non-action, making a *best decision*, is priceless.

In summary, from a universal perspective, the sole purpose of non-action is to maintain present moment focus – which innately enhances inner vitality, connection to the wisdom of the soul, and magnetically draws appropriate experiences to us (in the form of people, objects and events). The outcome of non-action, presence, is enhanced dreams, intuition, and synchronicity. We tap in to heightened consciousness (including the *stream of consciousness*). By connecting to the core aspect of self and consciousness, we tap into an innate *sixth sense*. This helps us see things more clearly, helps us make better decisions, and *magnetically* (energetically) attracts appropriate opportunities that in the long-run best match our core truth.

The Tao states that the *common* person is forever *doing* (taking as-though-random direct action) – and yet leaves much incomplete (undone). In contrast, the master is forever *being* (engaged in non-action) and thereby is said to leave nothing undone. The master practices non-action and thereby attracts appropriate experience. Similarly, due to a constant practice of non-action, the master is described as *being* able to teach without speaking and affecting the world without leaving home. We draw appropriate experience merely by being.

When in a state of being (i.e., present-moment mindfulness), we do not have a specific goal. We allow the flow of the present moment's connection to core truth to guide us. The Tao paradoxically states in seemingly backward fashion that when we have no goal – i.e., when we are present – all our (direct) actions shall succeed. The reasons for this are twofold. First, by focusing in the present moment we are guided to appropriate experience. Second, lack of expectation enhances probability of a successful result – as expectation infers so-called future focus, indicating focus in the ego – which is not connected to core truth and so suggests expectation of a less-than-appropriate experience, which may become a self-fulfilling (as though prophetic) outcome.

Non-action is subtle. Yet powerful. Its essence is intangible. Yet its results are material and, at times, monumental. The Tao states that the ethers of non-action, although negligible in space and substance, are able to permeate even the region of zero space – effecting change anywhere and everywhere.

ACTION – RIGHT ACTION

Long ago I was graced with an invitation to meditate in the home of Tibetan Lama Arjia Rinpoche in Mill Valley, California. I observed his every movement and tried to understand his approach to life. My impression was that in every moment, Lama Rinpoche silently asks himself: *"What is right action in this moment?"* – i.e., what is the best action I can take in this moment? And this moment. And this moment. Ad infinitum.

> *When you [attempt to] stop activity to attain quietude,*
> *your very effort fills you with activity.*
>
> *Deny the reality of things*
> *and you miss their reality.*
>
> *The more you talk and think about [truth],*
> *the further you wander from truth.*
>
> *[This is not right activity.]*
>
> *To return to the root is to find the essence,*
> *but to pursue appearances or* enlightenment
> *is to miss the Source.*

> *Hsin-hsin Ming* (*Verses on the Faith Mind*)
> by Seng-Ts'an, Third Zen Patriarch

When living in Sausalito, California, a gorgeous Mediterranean-like, mountainous, seaside town built upon a busy harbor system, I had the good-fortune to befriend Vince and Gloria DiBiase. I first met Gloria while she worked in the ***Tibetan Culture House*** shop in San

Rafael. The store was packed full of colorful goods from Tibet, Nepal, and India. Gloria and I spoke for an hour upon meeting while I tried on a few garments and asked questions regarding traditional Tibetan objects that I had not seen before. At the conclusion of our conversation she mentioned that she felt that her husband and I are of seemingly like-mind and like-heart, and suggested that we meet sometime. A few weeks later I met Vince.

Vince DiBiase was born in New York City. Vince met Gloria in 1972 and moved to San Francisco in February of 1974 to catch the latter aspect of the sixties movement in its glory at its mecca – San Francisco. Vince and Gloria loved nature and, after giving a ride to a young female hitch-hiker who gave them a tour of Marin County, moved to this gorgeous area. The southern perimeter of Marin County is a scenic, fifteen-minute drive from the urbanity of San Francisco, yet secluded with thick forest on the side of Mount Tamalpais. During the sixties the area was chock full of mainstream *drop-outs* who sought a more creative and purposeful existence. Many significant musical groups recorded albums here – including Fleetwood Mac, Santana, The Grateful Dead, Janis Joplin, Quicksilver Messenger Service, etc. As Vince describes it, "Marin County was 'Middle Earth' [back then]."

I was introduced to Vince at Sweetwater Saloon, a then-renowned music venue in Mill Valley. Moments after meeting, Vince invited me for a walk outside the bar. He told me that he moved to San Francisco to experience the tail-end of the sixties movement, but also wanted to gain access to the study and practice of holography – a technological art form that was co-birthed in 1974 at Stanford University, in Palo Alto. By the mid-seventies, Vince had become a *third-wave* holographer, practicing the art form/science. He opened a holography studio in San Rafael that was open to the public.

In 1983, while managing Holos Gallery, a holography gallery in SF (one of four in the country), a manager of the Grateful Dead saw a bumper sticker hologram on Vince's car promoting the film *ET*. The manager told Vince that the Grateful Dead might be interested in similar merchandising of their brand name using holograms. At the time, the holograms were being distributed with *Mars* candies. Vince designed holography merchandising for the Grateful Dead which was well received by the manager. But before the program was approved, the manager left the band.

After a while, Jerry Garcia spoke directly with Vince regarding holograms. Although Jerry and Vince had not yet met in-person, Jerry invited Vince to a few of his band's shows. Finally after a few years of communication, Vince met with Jerry to present holograms. Garcia loved the forms. More so, Garcia found that he and Vince had much in common. So much that they became close friends. Vince mentioned his amazement at Garcia's scope of interest, which included holography and nanotechnology, in addition to his obvious prowess as musician and artist. Their friendship blossomed quickly and effortlessly due to almost daily contact – as Gloria, Vince's wife, had become the daily, full-time nanny of Jerry's daughter, Keelin. Vince would drop Gloria at Jerry's in the morning, and pick her up every evening. Typically, Vince and Jerry would connect for a bit in the evenings, when Vince picked up Gloria. Gloria traveled to distant Grateful Dead shows and vacations with Jerry, his daughter Keelin, and Keelin's mother, Menasha. Eventually Jerry invited Vince to join Gloria and Jerry's family on the road. Jerry then asked Vince if he would handle personal business ventures for him – namely, real estate and his budding art and clothing businesses.

In December of 1992, Jerry attended a successful gallery exhibition of his art that Vince had coordinated. Gloria continued to serve as the family's caretaker and also found Jerry's final home – a lovely 4-bedroom house with a view of San Francisco Bay. On Cinco de Mayo (the Fifth of May, the Mexican holiday) in 1995, Jerry's wife, Deborah, terminated Vince and Gloria – for reasons that were unclear. Perhaps she simply wanted more private time with her husband. Three months later, the evening before his premature passing, Jerry went to dinner with Deborah at a local restaurant. They had a vigorous disagreement during the meal. Jerry didn't return home but, rather, checked into a rehab center just west of Fairfax – which didn't have an MD on staff. He died in the early morning hours. Vince and Gloria were shocked that their friend had passed.

Approximately three years later, Vince met Tibetan lama Arjia Rinpoche, who lived with his extended family in nearby Mill Valley. The lama was creating a 3-dimensional mandala – and learned that

Vince was proficient with holography. The lama asked to meet Vince as he considered development of a hologram of the mandala.

The lama and Vince quickly bonded and Vince subsequently served as the lama's secretary for three years. During the initial six months of service, Vince didn't realize the magnitude of the lama's position, responsibilities, reputation, and international stature. At this time, the lama asked Vince to review an article in *U.S. World News and Report* which mentioned the lama. The article described the esteemed status of the lama. [Author's Note: Arjia Rinpoche is largely responsible for the practice and evolution of Tibetan Buddhism in the USA. He now lives in Bloomington, Indiana, where he is director of the Tibetan Mongolian Buddhist Cultural Center and Kumbum Chamtse Ling Temple.]

The next morning, Vince apologized to the lama – as their relationship was quite informal, consisting of much joking, etc. After reading the article, Vince asked whether he should bow to the lama and formalize his conduct when in his presence. The lama accepted Vince's apology yet suggested that he preferred that their relationship remain informal by stating, "That's okay, we are friends."

Vince and the lama spent much time together. Vince answered many questions regarding the English language – which supported the lama's use of a Tibetan/Chinese–English pocket-translator. And Vince helped the lama create literature (brochures, cards, flyers, etc.). Vince noted that for every suggestion that he would present to the lama regarding the use of Photoshop software, by the next morning the lama would work with the software and present ten suggestions to Vince. In other words, Vince realized that despite a language barrier that the lama was exceptionally bright and resourceful, while maintaining a behind-the-scenes personality that loved to joke and laugh.

Shortly after my initial meeting with Vince, he suggested I visit the lama at his home. He arranged for me to meditate with the lama and a small group of devotees on a Sunday morning and a weekday evening.

On a crisp Sunday morning, Vince and I drove through the elegant town of Mill Valley and crept up the foothills of Mt. Tamalpais, eventually making our way to the winding single-lane road that led to the door of the lama's home. The setting was subtly exquisite as the two-story home is quietly nestled away from the road in such way that it is all but hidden amid thick brush and redwoods. A wisp of white smoke curled from the crimson-red chimney, bent to leeward by the early-morning breeze, gently meandering through the top of the canopy of shorter foliage and past enormous torsos of the trunks of numerous majestic redwood trees. In other words, the scene was as beautiful as I had ever seen — a pristine, post-card moment.

At the door we were met by a beautiful woman with young child in tow, both wearing colorful, draped linens. She welcomed us into the home. It was obvious that she held high regard for Vince. A dozen Tibetan figures were dashed about the home, preparing food in the kitchen, setting the dining table, laughing and chatting in the living room, and meditating upstairs. Each held a quiet warmth and sincere gaze upon meeting. Vince led me to a stairway near the kitchen that led to a small rehabbed attic space. The attic meditation room, with A-frame ceiling, accommodated a group of twenty students who sat in meditation waiting for the lama and his protégé to join the weekly ceremony. I made my way through the array of seated meditators and found a zafu to sit upon. I closed my eyes, took a few deep abdominal breaths, and did my best to let go of all thoughts and anticipation, for I knew that only by focusing in the moment could I gain entry into the aspect of the moment that is typically hidden.

Ten minutes later, Lama Rinpoche joined us. He appeared much like the revered Dali Lama — close to his age, size, and similar in appearance. Certainly he appeared as described — *the intellectual lama*. His protégé was twenty years old, thin, with shaved head and obvious curiosity that caused him to look about the room; he made eye contact with his obvious many friends, all the while smiling. He did not carry himself with the *all-business* earnestness of his teacher, a welcome relief. Little did I know that the lama, too, had a great sense of humor and expressive joy — but that would only be seen later, outside the confines of the morning ritual.

The lama sat in front of us, with his protégé at his side. Initially they both kneeled in front of us, kneeling before the Buddha, with hands clasped first over the crown of the head, then in front of the third eye (between the brows), then before the heart, and then they bent to the floor with palms still clasped at the level of the heart. They did this numerous times before taking their places on zafus at the front of the room, facing the group of meditators. We followed their every action. First, we meditated. Then we chanted. Then Lama Rinpoche shared thoughts regarding life for half an hour. Then we ate. Over time I learned more about the lama. He seemed very bright yet surprisingly simple. My impression was that in every moment he recited an inner mantra: "What is right activity [in this moment]?" *He then followed the guidance of his inner voice. Always.*

Right activity is aligned with the voice of the soul and universal consciousness. Consciousness speaks to us through enhanced dreams, intuition, and synchronicity [See *Voice of the Soul: A Call to Action*, Volume Three in the Anatomy of the Human Fabric trilogy, for further explanation]. Inner guidance is accessed through soul-aligned activity (including the ultimate soul-aligned activity – namely, stillness meditation). The soul's guidance directs the self to two types of activity in any given moment. Direct activity and non-activity. **Right activity in any moment, whether direct or passive, creates the highest benefit in the long-run on all levels of being (at the levels of the personality, soul, and oversoul) for all beings.**

Direct activity is externally-directed activity that directly supports accomplishment of a material agenda. Non-activity is described as internally-directed activity that supports personal well-being and long-term benefit (enhanced energetic vibration) at the soul level— which serves to attract appropriate experience in the form of people, objects, and events that will serve to trigger appropriate lessons.

As an example of right action, consider an individual who is having difficulty deciding what topic to study in college. The answer may be accessed through the inner voice (dreams, intuition) and supported by external signs (synchronicity). Enhanced dreams, intuition, and synchronicity are developed through non-activity – activities that are intended solely to enhance presence (the creative womb of self-awareness, self-evolution, and the supportive experiences necessary to bring forth awareness through mastery of fundamental life lessons).

Non-activity (*being*) lifts internal awareness and reveals one's unique life purpose and life service. In this example, once inner and external signs have guided the person to knowing what topic to study, the person employs direct activity such as enrolling in the curriculum, paying intuition, buying books, and studying – to accomplish the material aspect of the task at hand. Right action is the application of appropriate non-activity in every moment and, at times, is appropriate direct activity. [Again, see *Voice of the Soul: A Call to Action* for a detailed explanation of non-action.]

ACTIVITY (THOUGHT, WORD, AND ACTION)

Activity is comprised of thought, word and action. Thought includes intention. Word is spoken expression, including toning and mantra (phonetics). Action includes both outward expression, direct action intended to influence a material outcome, and non-action which intends (and supports) present moment focus, via inner effect – as discussed earlier in this text.

Activity is aligned with either the soul (conscious activity) or with the ego (unconscious activity), in each moment. One or the other. This is a choice we make in each moment: whether to align with ego or soul. The definitive signs of soul alignment are receipt of enhanced dreams, intuition, and synchronicity. And concurrent focus in the present moment. [See *Voice of the Soul: A Call to Action* for an in-depth discussion of how to align with soul ... or ego.]

ANTAHKARANA

The Antahkarana is our energetic template. It succinctly describes how we evolve. Thus it is the template of human transformation. The Antahkarana is described in detail in *Voice of the Soul: A Call to Action*. The Antahkarana is comprised of two functional elements. First, the Line of Force is an energetic cord that theoretically reaches from Heaven to (the center of the) Earth via the precise energetic centers (of each of the seven major chakras) of a human being. Second, Spheres of Influence, vortex-like cords that connect to this Line of Force, extend to every corner of the Universe. The Spheres of Influence look like the cords that extend from a maypole or tetherball court. They connect us to people, objects and events (the building-blocks of experience – wherein appropriate experience triggers us to evolve).

Evolution is objectively defined (measured)
By the degree of verticality and girth of one's Line of Force.

Jesus Christ, the Buddha, Allah, Krishna, and Mohammad each had a perfectly vertical Line of Force of tremendous width (radii); like a river of energy the energies of Heaven and Earth flowed through them — energizing and inspiring these great beings to serve as conduits of Heaven and Earth. In comparison, we mortal humans have a line of force which is neither perfectly vertical nor of great radius. *Wherever the Line of Force is kinked (not vertical, i.e., with horizontal skew), we hold unresolved issues in subconscious and conscious aspects of our being. So,* **the purpose of experience is to straighten (verticalize) the Line of Force at every point where it is kinked. And as we verticalize the Line of Force, it naturally gains strength and increasing radius — influencing greater connection to the wisdom and energy of Heaven and Earth. The relative verticality and girth of one's Line of force is a barometer of their evolution.**

Spheres of influence are connectors to the building blocks (props) of experience. The props of experience are people, objects, and events. They serve to trigger us to again feel emotions that we were not ready to resolve — which **must** be re-experienced (re-felt) to be healed.

Summation. How does the mechanism of the Antahkarana function? Like cords on a maypole, Spheres of Influence connect to specific people, objects, and events – the props of experience, to connect us to a necessary experience that will trigger an opportunity to evolve (by triggering us to re-feel previously buried emotion which, this time around, we can choose to appropriately process, release, and heal/ evolve — or we can again choose to avoid appropriately processing the emotion and can again bury the unresolved emotion in our subconscious energetic template). The Spheres of Influence bring the energy of the experience to the Line of Force — which holds the unresolved subconscious energy. How we choose to process the experience effects the Line of Force. If we appropriately process and release the prior unresolved energy, the Line of Force removes the horizontal kink that represented the unresolved energy (and thus verticalizes the Line of Force where before there was the unresolved horizontal kink).

Again, the verticality and girth of the Line of Force provides an objective indication of one's degree of evolution.

ATTRACTION – THE LAW OF ATTRACTION

The reason we exist is to evolve. Our ultimate purpose is to learn about ourselves — i.e., gain self-awareness. To learn we must master life lessons. So ... we as-though-magnetically *attract* perfectly appropriate, perfectly timed life experiences.

NOTE

We are *holistic* beings. This, simply defined, means that we are comprised of a body and mind — and that body and mind are intimately entwined (connected). So, in essence we are a *bodymind*. To learn in complete fashion — to acquire mastery of the self — we must engage **both** body and mind. Thoughts are located in the brain (mind). Emotions — *the body's response to the mind's thoughts* — are located in the body (according to the ancient Taoists, more specifically in the internal organs). Whereas the (conscious) mind learns through spoken and written word — the body (i.e. bodymind) learns through *experience.* This is why *hands-on* training is more effective than training merely through (off-site) reading or explanation. We transform the subconscious energetic template through *experience.* We transform the shadow — the unresolved aspect of the egoic personality — through experience. Knowledge is information accumulated in the conscious mind (through reading, etc.). Wisdom is knowledge that has been integrated into the body through *experience*.

(end of NOTE)

To master lessons, we engage experiences that challenge the unresolved aspects of the self. Resolution of the unresolved (wounded) aspects of self *is* evolution. We *must* experience to evolve; i.e., we do not evolve via thinking. Further, we must be challenged by appropriate experiences — i.e., by experiences that serve to teach us lessons that we need to learn. So, how do we *find* appropriate *learning* experiences? We attract them.

Our inner energy, comprised of subconscious and conscious energetic templates, draws appropriate *learning* experiences to us — that will help us resolve unresolved *issues;* in technical energetic terms, we must release/tonify vibrational stagnancies in the Antahkarana's Line of Force (as explained in the section entitled Antahkarana, we must make the Line of Force more vertical, and thereafter increase the girth of the Line of Force). Experiences are carried to us by triggers — appropriate (specific) people, objects, and events. These triggers (people, objects, and events) cause us to react at a core level — emotionally and/or mentally. To evolve (heal) we must *re-feel* unresolved, buried emotions. Unresolved emotions must be revealed to heal (similar to how a pimple must release buried pus to heal) ...

> *To heal unresolved emotion previously buried*
> *in the recesses of the subconscious aspect,*
> *we must reveal, re-feel and release*
> *the unresolved emotion/energy*
> *from the bodily aspect of the bodymind.*
> [See *Emotional Release.*]

The wounded aspect of our inner energetic template radiates like a magnet, transmitting a message to appropriate people, objects, and events that will challenge us — drawing them to us — so we (and they) can resolve.

The mechanism of the law of attraction magnetically draws triggers (people, objects, and events) that will cause us to re-experience and even magnify the intensity of the unresolved emotion/thoughts that we are experiencing. For example, if we are dealing with unresolved anger — we will attract triggers that cause us to experience even greater anger. Sorry if that's not what you wanted to hear! If we are dealing with unresolved sadness, we draw people, objects, and events that cause us to experience enhanced sadness. Why?

Healing Crisis:
A gift of extraordinary proportion
from the perspective of the soul.

The reason we attract triggers that enhance our experience of unresolved emotions/thoughts is to force us to undergo a *healing crisis*. How does a healing crisis help us? The overwhelming discomfort of a healing crisis motivates us to heal — so as to minimize the discomfort (preferably ASAP). Earlier, we might not have been inspired to heal, as we were not exceptionally uncomfortable. A healing crisis inspires us to face the issues, gain understanding, and resolve subconscious and conscious wounds. Healing crises are commonplace (i.e., are apparently a necessary aspect of the human condition) — as it is only the rare individual that chooses to confront and resolve core energetic conflict in the absence of necessity (i.e., without being confronted with the discomfort of healing crises).

As a summary, The Law of Attraction serves to enhance our mastery of life lessons. We attract triggers (in the form of people, objects, and events) that dig up buried wounds by triggering us to re-experience and react to previously unresolved core emotion/thought. When necessary we attract uncomfortable situations, healing crises, to inspire us to evolve.

BLAME

If we blame another, there is no end to blame. Blame begets more blame. Blame is conduct of the egoic aspect of personality (*monkeymind*). Ego never takes responsibility for its own actions. Soul never blames another for its own actions. Soul always looks at the self, and recognizes what we contribute to any situation. If another person hurts us, it's our responsibility to resolve the situation — either by working through the issue with the other party (if they are open to the process of resolution), or by exercising discernment that prescribes walking away (especially if an abusive situation). Blame fails to realize that the other party to any dynamic is merely a mirror reflection of the self. As adults, we consent to be in any situation. If in an abusive situation – exercise discernment and get out of harm's way ASAP. In any other non-abusive circumstance, consider how you are responsible for the situation. Do not blame the other. Look at yourself. Consider how your thoughts, words and/or actions contributed to the situation.

BODY – MAINTENANCE OF THE PHYSICAL BODY

The foundation of an efficient self-healing regimen is comprised of proper nutrition, exposure to sunshine, positive thought, and minimized stress-related reactivity. Healthful practices such as yoga, qi gong (t'ai chi), physical exercise, conscious creativity (creating via the five physical senses – such as creating visual art, music, dance, etc. – while experiencing real-time emotion, in the moment), self-expression, and other disciplines support self-healing. Three types of *conscious activity* (body-centered breathing, expression via the five senses, and reception via the five senses) access the wisdom of the soul – via enhanced dreams, intuition, synchronicity, and miracles – to reveal life purpose and life service. [Note: A detailed discussion of soul-aligned activity is found in *Voice Of The Soul: A Call To Action.*]

Energy (Sanskrit – *prana*, Chinese – *chi* and *shen*) is most easily assimilated through simpler ways of being – such as exposure to fresh air, sunlight, bathing in seawater, and ingestion of vegetable and nut food groups. *Lack of energetic vitality results from inappropriate conditions of living – including inappropriate thought focus and misuse of food.*

The ancients discovered that there is a direct correlation between the potency of prana (energetic fluids) and the ability of an individual to become more sensitive (attuned) to progressively subtle ethereal energies. To this effect, an esoteric group of Tibetans proposed that those casually engaged in the quest for enhanced self-awareness may eat whatever foods they so choose, including meat – until such time as the individual begins to experience, and pursue, ever-heightening self-awareness. As one becomes more sensitive certain restrictions to diet *may* be helpful. The progressively sensitive person *might* consider a vegetarian diet.

The esoteric Tibetans claim that this rule may not be violated once a certain juncture on the path (of personal evolution) is achieved. Vegetables, grains, fruits, and nuts are suggested fare. Eggs and cheese may be included in the diet – however, these may hinder those in the process of developing psychic abilities; hence, no eggs and minimal cheese are advised. The Tibetans classify milk and butter under a separate grouping such that they may be consumed.

As an example, the esoteric ancient Tibetans believe that those who have maintained a long-term, strict vegetarian diet may effectively engage in extrasensory activity. Specifically, they believed that only individuals who were strictly vegetarian for ten years could *effectively* read the *Akashic Record* (an aspect of what Carl Jung described as the Collective Conscious – an energetic record of history transcending time and space). They felt that these are the only restrictions regarding diet.

Other attributes that profoundly affect the physical aspect of the bodymind are **common sense and senses of compassion, humor, and faith**. The esoteric Tibetans felt that these are our greatest assets. Common sense understands that progress takes time – it is seldom instantaneous. The esoteric Tibetans claim that abstinence from meat, nicotine, and alcohol, when aligned with a relatively disciplined life, will induce the Pineal Gland to highest endocrine/energetic function, furthering higher connection. Paradoxically, note that unless the intention behind maintenance of a vegetarian diet is in accordance with one's (higher) path, then the aforementioned diet is of little use; in other words, if someone does not eat meat only because they do not like the flavor of meat, their intention of vegetarianism is not in accord with the *spirit of vegetarianism*, which honors animal life, and thereby such an intention does not further personal self-awareness (evolution).

Fresh air, sunlight, minimized stress, and positive thoughts help to create a healthy physical body (bodymind). Fresh air carries negative ions with reductive (anti-oxidant) properties. **Body-centered breath-**

ing profoundly enhances the energy of the physical body. [See *Voice of the Soul: A Call to Action*].

The energy of the sun may be safely harnessed to vitalize our energy by using specific methods (e.g., a qi gong blinking method described by Mantak Chia). Minimization of stress helps the body in obvious ways. Positive thought is essential to the efficient functioning of the human body (and energetic system). Positive thought may be bolstered by silent and/or spoken affirmations and indirectly supported by energetic disciplines (such as yoga, qi gong, meditation, and conscious creative expression). The Taoists believe that *what we focus upon in the moment is all that we are*, for the present moment is all that exists. Focus upon positivity begets affirmative physical manifestation.

BODY LANGUAGE

Body posture speaks loudly. A smile, a frown, crossed arms, crossed legs, a raised eyebrow, hands held as fists, arms held wide open, and one's coming a bit too close, have obvious meaning.

Another type of body language, albeit seemingly subtle – yet powerful – concerns our bodily relationship to another, with related *energetic (including chakra-to-chakra) positioning*. In this way and others, people unknowingly play energy games.

NOTE

The chakras (see the chapter entitled *Chakras*) are energetic vortices, funnel-like in shape, that extend from our vertical center-line both forward and backward. Seven major chakras range vertically in position from the perineum (groin) to the crown of the head.

A person may unknowingly try to *take* energy from another person (when feeling insecure or when trying to dominate/control the other). The method? Person A stands directly in front of Person B while engaging them. In other words, Person A's chakras exactly face (and overlap) Person B's chakras. Again, this is a very subtle dynamic – yet the effects are noticeable. How can you test this theory? By consciously avoiding this dynamic. Specifically, if ever confronted by a individual (perhaps a boss, a dominant/controlling person, or an insecure/victim-like person) who stands (or sits) directly in front of you – with their shoulders directly squaring-off to your shoulders while facing one another – then move your torso so it does not exactly square-off to them. You will notice they react by turning so they again precisely squared-off to you. Why? When squared-off, the dominant or insecure person feels *stronger* – as though usurping energy from the other individual's energy system. In this dynamic, Person A also may be standing *a bit too close* to Person B. So, take a step or two back, and turn a bit away from squared-off position, to defuse the chakra-to-chakra dynamic.

While working in energywork and bodywork in table-based sessions as a healing practitioner – with clients lying horizontal on a massage table (on their backs, fully-clothed) – I am careful not to square-off with the central vertical (a.k.a. Central Channel or Antahkarana Line of Force) energy meridians and chakras of clients. In other words, if I am sitting near the head of the person, at the end of the table, I am certain not to sit with my torso's center-line blocking the energetic line of their Crown (7th) and Central Channel or Antahkarana Line of Force. (To do so, I sit at an angle at the end of the table, and/or a bit to one side of the table), even if only a few inches from the centerline.

(end of NOTE)

BODYMIND

The body holds only (conscious) answers.
The mind holds only questions.

Anonymous

Holistic theory and practice, by definition, view body and mind as a single, unified unit. Body and mind so intimately affect one another that they are best considered as an integral unit. For example, the brain affects the body via the endocrine (hormone) system – sending chemical messengers through the blood stream – that inspire activity in the body. The brain also sends messages to the body via the nervous system (motor nerves). The body affects the mind – sending continual messages to the brain – via sensory nerves and biochemical feedback. Body and mind communicate with, and affect, one another via various chemical and neurological processes in such intimacy that they are, functionally, one inseparable unit.

Note that whereas Western psychology treats the emotions as though nothing more than mental substrates, presumably located in the brain, Eastern psychology considers the emotions to be bioenergetic substrates that are stored in specific internal organs. Eastern psychology (psychoenergetics) states that *emotions are the body's response to thought*, stressing the strength of the body/mind connection.

BODYWORK

Bodywork is simply that. It influences inner energetic meridians, which impact physicality, mentality, emotionality, and spirituality. Reception of kinesthetic attention may have profound healing effect – healing both conscious and subconscious aspects of one's being. [See *Voice of the Soul: A Call to Action*].

BREATH

> *Breath is the bridge to Consciousness.*
>
> Anonymous

Breath is comprised of both physical and energetic components. *Physical breath* moves *air* into and from the lungs via inhalation and exhalation. *Energetic breath* moves the *energy of air* (prana) into and from the body's energy systems. Energetic breath (energy of air) is moved via mental focus (intention) and physical expression of the body (for example, diaphragmatic movement causes movement of the energy of the air throughout the torso). Body-centered energetic breathing accesses heightened consciousness by connecting the bodymind to the wisdom and vitality of Heaven and Earth.

We can affect our health and state of being (degree of consciousness) by employing body-centered breathwork. An example is *Abdominal Breathing* – a simple yet challenging technique that helps the bodymind to ground (take rootedness in the energy of the Earth) and center (strengthening the Antahkarana/Central Channel of energy that extends infinitely upward and downward to anchor us in Heaven and Earth energies). The technique of abdominal breathing requires mental focus upon the rise and fall of the lower abdomen (specifically, the Lower Tan T'ien – a powerful energy center located three inches below the navel in the centerline of the lower torso). This serves to bring energy of the breath (energy of air – light, prana, shen, etc.) to the Lower Tan T'ien, which invigorates the body, especially connecting us to grounding energy of the Earth, and defeats the scattered wanderings of the monkeymind's focus upon distraction. The Lower Tan T'ien is an incredibly powerful energy center – so powerful that (of course) this is where a zygote develops into an infant, at the center of the womb. Of course we nourish children in a profoundly powerful area of the body – to best support the infant's physical and energetic development.

The power of prayer, intention, and activity is exponentially enhanced when coupled with a foundation of body-centered (conscious) breathing, as conscious breath helps complete a *grounded* and *centered* circuit that spans Heaven and Earth. This serves to turbo-charge prayer, intention, and activity.

BUSINESSPERSON

The best businessperson serves the communal good, and thereby herself. Plans that consider long-term scenarios not only optimize community benefit, but tend to maximize income in the long-run.

The best businessperson is aware that two types of income exist – financial income and psychic income. Psychic income benefits all aspects of life other than the pocketbook. Psychic income is the ancillary value that is derived from a job. Psychic income enhances happiness, joy and/or bliss. For example, psychic income derived from working in a coffee shop might include enjoyable conversations with patrons and networking benefits. Psychic income derived from working aboard a ship might include being outdoors on the sea, seeing distant ports of call, meeting foreign people, etc. Total income associated with a business venture includes both financial and psychic income.

A wise employer of personnel treats employees as though family – as any business is only as good as its employees. Employees are inspired to perform highest-caliber services if treated with respect and given reasonable compensation for their effort.

CAREER

What we do for a living is of little importance if considered from the perspective of the soul. What matters is that we consciously (i.e., with loving awareness) participate in every moment, regardless of the task at hand. Give from the depth of your heart and act impeccably – in all moments. No matter what is asked of you. No human being is better than any other human being. No job is better than any other job. All jobs are necessary. It is better to be a janitor with an openly loving heart than to be a brain surgeon with a closed heart.

However, *each soul on the planet has a unique life purpose and life service.* [For detailed explanation, see *Voice of the Soul: A Call to Action.*] As such, certain jobs allow us to express these specific talents and missions more easily than do other jobs. So, although it is both honorable and valuable to maintain an open heart (and energy systems) while engaged even in menial work, it is beneficial to maintain a career that supports ultimate expression of one's unique, soul-aligned talents. Jobs appropriate for our vibration allow us to grow (i.e., most efficiently and effectively learn and gain mastery of appropriate life lessons), help us to remain open-hearted regardless of activity, and help us to most completely serve others.

CARING

Eastern philosophy believes that the great Tao, the force that creates and empowers all of creation, is the foundation of all. Thus, s/he who directly cares about the Tao indirectly cares about all things. To be caring is to maintain humility and reverence before the Tao and, thus, before all animate beings and inanimate things. A profoundly caring relationship engages mutual caring between partners based upon an innate foundation of mutual caring for the Tao (and thereby, again, all beings).

CHAKRA

Chakra is a Sanskrit term which translates to *spinning wheel*. There are seven major chakras in the bodymind. They range in position from the perineum (groin) to the crown of the head. Each progressively higher-positioned chakra spins at a higher velocity. Each chakra represents a distinct aspect of the human condition. For example, the first chakra, the Root Chakra, energetically describes safety issues; the second chakra represents sexual, reproductive, and creative issues. The third chakra, the Solar Plexus Chakra, represents masculinity, power, issues of the personal will and ego. The fourth chakra, the Heart Chakra, represents loving connection to others; the fifth chakra, the Throat Chakra, represents communication — externally expressing our truth, and internally hearing the inner voice; the sixth chakra, the Third Eye, represents extrasensory perception and connection, including telepathy. The seventh major chakra, the Crown Chakra, represents our connection to the Universe.

The health of the chakras is diagnosed through the strength and direction of their spin. Clockwise spin (for those born in the Northern Hemisphere) represents vitality. Counter-clockwise spin represents vitality for those born in the Southern Hemisphere.

Each chakra corresponds to a specific color and musical tone (the colors of the rainbow, beginning with red, correspond to the first through seventh chakras, respectively; and the musical tones C through B correspond to the first through seventh chakras.

Expression and reception of activity via the five senses — via taste, smell, movement, vision and hearing (a.k.a. conscious-aligned activity) may heal the chakras. [See *Voice of the Soul: A Call to Action* for more information. Many books describe the chakras.]

CHANGE

Change is inevitable.

Everything changes — except the Absolute (i.e., natural order, God, etc.). Everything else is impermanent. Thus, she who is flexible and accepts change is a disciple of life. She who is rigid and resists change is a disciple of death.

Change is a great catalyst of transformation
as it pushes us into the ocean of uncertainty,
the great teacher
of Faith, of Patience, of Courage.

Change takes time. Profound and lasting personal transformation (i.e., inner change) takes time. The Ninety-Day Rule (see the section on *Timing*) specifies that profound and lasting change at the level of the subconscious mind and energetic template — the Antahkarana — takes at least ninety days. Why is it best that intended change takes time — rather than being instantaneous? Because if we could change things as we always preferred, immediately, we would never need to learn the lesson of patience — as we would never need to wait for anything. Note that patience is one of the three great virtues espoused by the Tao (along with simplicity and compassion). *Graceful change requires mastery of patience.*

Change teaches faith. Patience is the ultimate test of faith. Patience is effortless if we accept that change is *good* and will lead to a positive outcome on some level (be it physical, mental, emotional and/or spiritual). To maintain such an optimistic perspective of change, we must have faith that we will be given exactly what we need, exactly when we need it (with regard to our highest evolution). The functional definition of faith is knowing that we are always perfectly provided for. Mastery of the lesson of graceful change requires mastery of faith.

Change teaches courage. To master change requires mastery of courage. Courage is defined as not allowing fear and doubt to thwart one's progress on an appropriate path. Courage inspires stepping through profound fear and doubt to accomplish an appropriate goal. Mastery of the lesson of graceful change requires mastery of courage.

Change is a catalyst of transformation. Without external change, we feel relatively comfortable — as conditions seem certain (temporarily). We are not externally *driven* to internal transformation when uncertain external conditions are gradual and gentle. In contrast, abrupt change in external conditions destabilizes a (temporary) sense of homeostasis, creating inner discomfort, which may inspire internal transformation (a.k.a. healing crisis).

In summation, change of external circumstances pushes us into uncertainty. External uncertainty activates doubt, worry, fear, anger, and/or anxiety (a combination of worry and anger). These feelings of emotion can seem quite powerful. Yet, if we so choose, our mentality — mental strength — can override even the most acute emotional discomfort. This is courage — the motivation to step through fear (and other stagnant emotionality). Courage is the choice to *do it anyway.* Only faith can cause us to summon the courage to step down the uncertain corridor. Faith in higher guidance and the probability of a preferred outcome may inspire us to move through change regardless how uncertain (and uncomfortable). Faith inspires patience. The soul is infinitely patient, as it maintains eternal faith — the soul is eternally aware that we are always taken care of; we are always given precisely what we need in any given moment (to learn now-relevant, appropriate lessons). In contrast, the ego demands instant gratification (i.e., is acutely impatient), as it holds not an iota of faith. Patience is the ultimate test of faith as only s/he who has faith may master the lesson of (graceful) patience. Change, a leap into the unknown, is a great teacher as it helps us to master essential life lessons (patience, courage, faith, release of emotional reactivity ... and more).

CLARITY

To see things as they are, we must see ourselves as we are. To see ourselves, we must be present. Focused only in this moment. Free of future expectation. Free of past attachments. Otherwise, we see everything through the tainted filter of our own unresolved energetic template and mis-color our perception of all externalities.

The quantum physicist's electron microscope alters the current position of an electron under scrutiny—such that truth, the true position of an electron, is altered by the viewer (a.k.a. seeker of truth).

The seeker of truth, through the explicit intention of seeking (an affirmation of incompleteness) and the action of seeking, alters truth. *Rather than seek truth, **be truth** (i.e., be present). This is clarity.* True (pure) clarity is innate when one accesses the present moment. *All externalities and internal functions may be clearly seen when we are present.*

Let things be as they truly are.
Accept.
Allow.
Let go of expectation.
Release attachment to outcome.
For then may we see clearly
and truly know
who we are
and the truth of all things.

Engage in conscious activity to develop clarity. Conscious activity creates immediate, innate (as-though automatic) focus in the present moment. [See *Voice of the Soul: A Call to Action.*] Clarity is a path of activity—comprised of thought (intention), word, and action that parallel the truth of your core being. Simply stated, to *intend* clarity is not enough as, like the quantum physicist, this serves merely to alter the natural course of things, pushing us away from clarity. We gain clarity through soul-aligned activity, not by seeking (or merely intending). Intention is not enough—the way of the spiritual warrior is a path of action, not thinking. Similarly, the path to clarity is through conscious action, not thinking.

For this reason, the paradox that is the *Tao Te Ching* states that if we look, we cannot see; and if we listen, we cannot hear. In other words, if we let go of the need to seek by instead simply engaging in our true nature in each moment (through soul-aligned activity), then truth may innately reveal itself.

25

Consider an analogy in which we are a muddy glass of water. Do you have the discipline to help the mud settle to the bottom (via practice of soul-aligned, conscious activity), leaving the water clear (i.e., rendering core truth)? [See *Voice of the Soul: A Call to Action.*]

COLLECTIVE CONSCIOUSNESS

A butterfly flutters its wings in Japan ...
a hurricane arises in the Azores.

Our energy affects others. This is obvious. But, perhaps what is not so obvious is that our energy affects *all* others and everything — including the Universe and Earth. As seemingly esoteric as this concept may seem, it holds great practical value.

It is obvious that our words and actions may affect others. If we focus a kind word or deed toward another, they are affected energetically (as manifested in physical, mental, emotional and/or spiritual form).

Less than obvious is the profound effect that our thoughts have upon others (and everything). Intention is powerful. Intention is the foundation of both word and action. Word and action arise only as a consequence of thought (intention). The Harvard Medical School studied the power of prayer on behalf of patients. Conclusion? Prayer works. Prayer tangibly supported the healing process of others. Surprisingly, a reputable center of the Western medicine confirmed that we are energetically connected!

Eastern philosophy believes that everything is inter-connected. Harvard Medical School's study on prayer supports this conclusion.

Quantum physics supports this theory, as atoms and subatomic particles permeate everything and thus are connected, indirectly, to all other atoms and particles. Interestingly, an electron looking through a room *sees* mostly empty space (99.9% of the space occupied by matter is atom-less but for the path of electron orbitals). So, from an electron's perspective, virtually everything looks the same and is connected by virtue of the relative vastness of empty space (and passing of an occasional electron and, more infrequently, other atomic particles).

The point is that since everything is interconnected, our thoughts are transmitted to everyone and everything. The interconnection of a Japanese butterfly (the *cause*) and Azorean hurricane (the *effect*) exemplifies the profound cause-and-effect mechanism that arises due to the unity of all beings and things.

The idea of a Collective Conscious (associated with a Stream of Consciousness) was presented, in part, to the mass Western culture by Dr. Carl Jung. He borrowed the concept from Eastern and indigenous philosophies. Ancients believed that the Stream of Consciousness consists of energetic threads, miniscule cords of light containing rivers of energy of comparatively diverse and distinct quality, that connect everything as though a great, seamless spider web through which energy (information) openly flows to-and-from everything in the Universe. (In the section, *Antahkarana*, above, these energetic tentacles are described as *Spheres of Influence*.) Anytime we effect change in our vibration we affect change in the vibration of the Collective as a whole, and each of its constituents. Further, esoteric philosophers believe that the Collective Consciousness (Stream of Consciousness) spans all (linear) time — connecting the present to so-called past and so-called future (more aptly in this understanding of reality, past and future do not exist, yet all moments may be accessed through the present moment when accessing the stream of consciousness).

COMMUNICATION

Become aware of your truth.
Then speak your truth completely.
Then be silent.

If thoughts are clear (regarding a preference, i.e., if you clearly know what you want), then *speak your truth completely and afterward be silent*, as all that needed to be communicated was stated. Only speak again when your thoughts are absolutely clear, if there is information that needs to be expressed to another party/parties. Or speak to clarify appropriate questions posed by the other party.

If thoughts are not clear (regarding a preference), then be silent while gaining clarity. To gain clarity, practice soul-aligned activity. [See sections entitled *Clarity* and *Action – Non-Action*.]

Dr. Fritz Perls, the founder of Gestalt Psychotherapy, advocated that the only candid statement is a *demand*, once one is clear with regard to what they want.

The purpose of communication is to express information to another party. In particular, the purpose of communication is to express information to another party, information (i.e., truth expressed in its highest essence) that serves to promote their highest evolutionary path (and thereby one's own highest path, the highest evolution of the Collective Conscious and universal consciousness).

Always express in a beneficial, loving way – in the kindest way possible considering the situation. If you cannot do so, respectfully tell the other party that you need time to collect your thoughts and/or resolve emotions that are blocking effective expression. Or, if appropriate due to time constraints, convey the information through a *safer* manner, perhaps by a written message (email, etc.) – which may evoke less emotion than any in-person expression – and offer a subsequent in-person meeting. Don't hide behind the veil of the internet, texting, or telephone – unless an in-person meeting might be abusive/unsafe. *Remember, there are lessons you are meant to learn from the other party.* An in-person meeting, even to discuss a breakup or firing, as awkward and difficult as it may be, may help both parties to resolve the lessons presented through the dynamic.

What information is beneficial? Any information that promotes the ultimate evolution of the other person. The truth is always beneficial, even if it isn't what the receiver wants to hear. BUT: if the details will unnecessarily *hurt* the receiver, then limit what you say to expressing only the basics (the essence of truth). For example, if breaking up or firing someone, it may be enough to inform the party that the relationship is terminated, and give a few essential elements of the explanation, without emotion. Be sensitive (empathic, sympathetic) and compassionate toward the other person. Be grateful that they came into your life—hard as this may be. Realize that they have helped you learn a necessary lesson, whatever that may be. And, that they too are simply human beings doing their best—whether or not you perceive their intention, words, and actions to be of value or not. So be respectful—always (unless the situation is abusive, then run, don't walk, out of harm's way).

Effective communication is *packaged* in a form that is most readily accessible from the perspective of the receiver. Say things in the kindest, most loving way possible—even when difficult. Don't sugar-coat truth. But also don't state non-essential details that will distract from processing the essence of truth. Don't *attack* the receiver—such information is never effectively *received* by the *defensive* receiver. Again, approach the receiver as gently and lovingly as possible. Always (again, unless in an abusive situation). Consider the timing of expression of information—ask the receiver when the best time might be to talk, per their timeframe, not yours.

Can one disclose too much information? Consider the extreme case of communicating with a child. Would you share all information with a child? No—as the child cannot process all information. Share information that serves to further the highest path of another party. Consider what's best for the other party to receive.

Is it necessary to share all facts that may be contrary to what another party prefers (e.g., in the case of a romantic or business rejection)? No. Be direct and firm, yet as gentle as possible, and tell the essence of the truth. Sharing all underlying details, which likely could be construed in a very negative light by the rejected receiver, might not be necessary to promote the receiver's best interest. Always tell the truth (in its highest essence). Never omit the highest essence of truth. But, again, underlying *hurtful* details may simply distract the best interest of the receiver.

When expressing, be certain not to convey facts in an emotional manner. In other words, don't dump your anger onto the receiver. This is not an appropriate release of emotion. [See *Voice of the Soul: A Call to Action* for explanation of *healthy* release of emotional energetic stagnancies.]

COMPASSION

Compassion, patience, and simplicity are the three great virtues.

Tao Te Ching

Namaste
From the Sanskrit:
"My soul recognizes your soul"
The foundation of compassion

Compassion is one of the three great virtues (along with patience and simplicity). To master compassion one must recognize that people have both an ego (profane, limited, unresolved aspect of personality) and soul. To have complete compassion we must learn how to rise above our own ego — and so access our soul. Only then can we clearly recognize another being's soul, and not simply view the other person as *their* ego (profane personality). Their soul, as ours, is flawless, infinitely-connected, and beautiful.

As an example, the term Namaste (or Jai Bhagwan) is understood to mean "my soul recognizes your soul." In other words, the intention is that "I do not view you through the egoic aspect of my personality" (and thereby see you as your limited egoic personality, which I may or may not *like* at the level of *personality*), but rather "I view you through my soul and see your soul — your beauty and humanity" — such that I may feel complete love and openness toward you. This is true compassion. In this way, Jesus, Muhammad, and the Buddha could feel complete love (i.e., compassion) for any person — regardless of their unresolved aspects. These great beings hold pure compassion. Before facilitating healing sessions, I was trained to repeat silently, "Jai Bhagwan (Namaste)" — to remind myself to view the other person as a soul, through my soul — and thereby to rise above the level of personality — so as to hold complete love, caring, and unity with other beings. To support access to my soul (i.e., access presence), I was taught to focus upon abdominal breathing. *In every moment.*

So, compassion is complete love and caring for another — regardless of the imperfection of the (egoic aspect of) personality as we — our

30

true self, our soul—recognize that the person's essence (true self) is his (her) soul, not flawed, limited personality.

Compassion is the key to forgiveness. For if we can see that another being, regardless how impaired, holds a beautiful soul—which we all do, as all souls are perfect—then we can feel complete love for that soul, and recognize that it is only the wounded aspect of his or her personality that has acted in a manner that is less than aligned with truth. In essence, we recognize and forgive the *human-ness* (mortality, finite nature, limited understanding) of the personality. This is true forgiveness—based upon true compassion.

CONFLICT

Your greatest nemesis
is your greatest teacher.

Those who inadvertently judge,
misuse or abuse,
serve us well
as they are a mirror reflection of our own shadow
and so teach us lessons about ourselves.

It is helpful to think of the other (resistant) party to a conflictive situation (a.k.a. the *adversary*) as a shadow that we ourselves cast. We attracted/created the situation. We drew the party and conflict to ourselves—to support our evolution. Their perspective serves as a mirror (or projection) of our own insecurities or inadequacies. We can observe and learn about an aspect of our *shadow* (ego-based) self by viewing all others—especially opposing/conflictive individuals. The great questions that arise in this perspective are: Why did we attract this resistant force? What unresolved lesson (that we have not yet consciously and subconsciously mastered) caused us to (subconsciously) attract the resistant force to us?

Recall that un-mastered lessons draw experiences/triggers (in the form of people, objects and events) that cause us to ultimately learn and master life's lessons. Try to learn what you can (about yourself) by studying the perspective of the resistant party. Try to resolve the issue in as kind and open a manner as possible. [See the section, *Communication*.]

Communicate with a resistant party only if you are absolutely clear regarding your thoughts and intention. If not clear, tell the party you need a bit of time to become clear, and practice soul-aligned activity [See the section on *Soul-Aligned Activity*, and, for a more detailed description, see *Voice of the Soul: A Call to Action*.]

Once thoughts and intention are clear (regarding preference), speak your truth completely, and then be silent. Wait patiently for a reply. If the reply is appropriate (logical, heart-felt, sincere), again speak only after thoughts are clear. If the reply is inappropriate, then either re-state your clear preference, or be silent (if you discern that the resistant party is incapable of effective communication and does not *comprehend* your statement or simply chooses to *resist* your statement). Consider telling them that you will be willing to open dialogue at a subsequent juncture, perhaps a couple months later — at which time you will be willing to clarify any questions they may have (to help them resolve lessons learned from your interpersonal dynamic). The idea here is that after an appropriate period of time, emotional reactivity of both parties will lessen, such that a healthy conversation may be possible, to help both parties learn the lessons presented by the dynamic. Examine the reason why you attracted this resistant party (a *trigger* for your own emotional reactivity). What unresolved inner wounds attracted this trigger (i.e., what unresolved wound needed to repeat this unresolved core lesson)?

Always be fair and generous when confronted with conflict (external or internal). Treat the resistant force as though a brother or sister. Listen completely to the resistant parties' words. Have compassion for their actions. Look at, and take responsibility for, your own emotional and mental reactivity. How did you contribute to the conflict? Don't simply run away — unless involved in an *abusive* dynamic — or both parties will miss the opportunity to learn the lesson at hand.

Rather than make the first move in any conflictive situation, it is better to observe the other party and await the appropriate time for movement. To this effect, the Tao says it is better to initially retreat a substantial distance than to move forward an inch. This innately enhances one's position without obvious assertive movement. By initially observing the other party, we gain information and, presumably, enhanced position, without physically imposing ourselves *against* the other party.

Never underestimate a resistant force. To do so is to all but guarantee defeat.

The very act of categorizing a resistant force as an *adversary* infers that her intention is *evil*. This is simply a mirror of our own unresolved issues (*evil* intention). The primary adversary is really our own unresolved woundedness. *It is our unresolved inner energies that attract an evil opponent to serve as a magnified reflection of our own unresolved psychenergy (also referred to as psychic energy).* Through this mechanism we are able to see just how unattractive and unenlightened our own unresolved reactivity may appear to be, as it is personified and illuminated through another's actions, helping us to gain realization that we should not behave that way. Oftentimes it is difficult to see our own *wounded attributes*, so we attract others with similar patterns of behavior to help us to visibly and obviously view our own unresolved behavior.

Neutralize *evil* by giving it nothing to oppose. If faced with what seems to be an *evil* force, do not actively engage with equal and opposite force. To do so is to act from ego, not soul, and will merely beget more of the same. Gain clarity (i.e., become aware of your truth). Then speak your truth (from the soul). Then be silent. By doing so, you do not oppose *evil* on its own terms, but rather, transcend the *evil* (by remaining aligned with your soul).

CONFUSION (LACK OF CLARITY AND CONFIDENCE)

When people lose their sense of wonder, they turn to religious authority (religion). When people cannot trust themselves, they turn to (governmental) authority. Knowing these tendencies, an astute leader helps people learn to trust themselves by guiding with a gentle and invisible hand. The people feel they are guiding themselves. [See the section entitled *Leadership*]. *As people gain trust in themselves, the need for authority subsides.* People's esteem increases. They then tend to engage in activities more aligned with their soul's core passion (soul-aligned activities, a.k.a. "conscious activity" — see the section entitled *Non-Action*). By doing so, they innately gain awareness of their true selves (life purpose and life service). Thus, the great leader steps back, to help diminish the confusion of the people. The great leader teaches through inspiration, leads by example, and so teaches without formal lessons. In this way, people let go of dependence upon the leader, and let go of the idea that the governor has knowledge greater than their own. Confusion dissolves. Clarity and confidence blossom.

CREATIVITY

True creativity seems simple, perhaps even juvenile, as it is beyond technique — as it is directly connected to Divine inspiration and intuition. True creativity soars beyond what seems possible, as in the music of Mozart, the art of Michelangelo, the dance of Baryshnikov. **True creativity is sourced by the soul of the artist/musician/dancer and is received by the soul of the observer.**

False creativity seems complex. It is merely technique-based and little more. False creativity is not sourced by the soul but, rather, by the ego. *False creativity may stimulate the ego of the observer, but it will not inspire their soul.*

The five senses are direct portals to the subconscious mind (and inner energetic template, the Antahkarana). This explains why creativity is essential to a balanced life. It accelerates our evolution. Creation while feeling real-time emotion accelerates release of unresolved psychenergy (psychic energy). [See *Voice of the Soul: A Call to Action* for detailed explanation.]

Core Mode of Expression. Every person is wired (born) as a dancer (athlete), visual artist, or musician. As a child, did you lose track of time more so when dancing (moving), drawing/painting, or expressing musically? This holds a clue regarding whether you're innately wired as a born dancer/athlete, artist, or musician. Certainly you may excel at more than one mode of core creative expression — nonetheless one primary mode of expression typically serves as the dominant trait.

Why is this important to identify? Your core mode of expression is an accelerated pathway to healing and evolving your subconscious mind and energetic core. For example, when you experience profound grief due to loss, you may benefit greatly by first engaging in daily cardiovascular-based movement, especially while feeling the emotions associated with grief. Such kinesthetic movement directly accesses the core energetic template (including subconscious mind), and accelerates release of emotion and other unresolved physical and mental energies. If you're wired from birth as a visual artist, then, when ready (after a period of days, weeks, or months), then augment your physical workouts (cardiovascular in nature) with creation of art based upon the real-time emotion you are feeling. This will further accelerate healing and evolution. If you're wired from birth as a musician, augment kinesthetic movement practice with creation of music, based upon real-time emotion (i.e., what you are feeling). If you are wired as a dancer/athlete, it is enough simply to create through dance and sport (while feeling real-time emotion).

Creativity, via the five senses, is a direct gateway to the subconscious mind, and entire inner energetic template (Antahkarana). Why is it important to create? *Primarily, as the process of creation (through the five senses) influences and heals the subconscious blueprint and, secondarily, as the vibration of the subconscious mind as-though-magnetically attracts our worldly experience.* The *Tao Te Ching* states that the Master "does without doing" (through practice of non-action). Creativity is a primary aspect of non-action—activity designed to enhance the vitality of our energetic template, which in turn serves to attract appropriate worldly experience.

When not feeling *creative*, move the body. You may find it easiest to create via the five senses if, beforehand, you vigorously move your body (and, as an aside, meditate). The reason? Full-body movement most quickly connects us to the energy of the Earth (grounding, rootedness). This helps defeat the scattered thoughts of the monkeymind and energizes the lower chakras, all of which helps us to feel more in tune with our true self—by connecting to the bodily aspect of bodymind. Daily repetition enhances the power of the movement. Full-body movement also serves to massage the internal organs, helping them release stagnant emotional psychenergy (psychic energy) [see the section entitled *Emotion*].

DEATH

If a person overcomes the fear of death, there is nothing that he (or she) cannot achieve—as in this fear itself has been transcended.

There are two major fears—primarily, fear of death and, secondarily, fear of loneliness. Presumably, one has transcended the fear of loneliness if they have transcended the fear of death. To conquer fear is to experience unconditional love (in every moment). When we experience unconditional love, we see truth. Including the truth of who we are, i.e., our life purpose and life service are clear. We accomplish all right activities. There is nothing *that is not right* that we cannot achieve.

For thousands of years, the Ancients have held the belief that an *enlightened* person may remain conscious during the process of dying—passing from physical form to energetic (soul) form. Obviously it is difficult to provide evidence to support this statement.

The death of a billionaire and the death of the wild animal, or insect, are the same with respect to universal impact. Death is death. Physical death is illusory. It is not an ending but, rather, simply a transition. So the soul of the billionaire, animal, and insect continue forward in a learning progression. All beings will ultimately attain enlightenment, given mastery of life lessons.

DECISIONS

All roads ultimately lead to the same place
as all roads teach life's lessons.
Yet specific roads more efficiently support our evolution.

What is most important is simply to *make a choice*. Take a reasonable amount of time to gain clarity regarding the pluses and minuses of options. If the options seem equally beneficial—it doesn't matter which option you select. Then, once reasonably clear, don't dawdle and procrastinate—make a decision and go for it. Give it all you've got! If the decision was not in your highest interest in any way, know that appropriate alternative doors of opportunity will open as you proceed, when appropriate. Why is this? Because the Tao knows precisely what lessons we need to master for our most efficient evolution. The Tao will provide the props of experience (appropriate people, objects, and events) that will help us to learn whatever life lessons we need to master for our personal evolution. If we make a less-than-appropriate decision, other doors of opportunity will open down the road—regardless what road you select. So ... all roads lead to the same place (i.e., to evolution and self-mastery)!

In the long run, it doesn't matter what you choose. It simply matters that you do choose—and then pursue that path. The Tao will do the rest (i.e., present alternative doors of opportunity if necessary for your evolution). Such understanding of the Tao is ... faith.

DEMAND

Fritz Perls, the so-called father of Gestalt psychotherapy, stated that the only honest statement, given clarity, is a demand. A demand is effectively presented with "I am clear that what I need is" as the introductory phrase. Once you are clear with what you need, a demand is the simplest, most direct, most concise mechanism by which to communicate. Inference that a statement is a demand does not mean that a harsh or hard tone of voice accompanies the statement. On the contrary, the gentler the tone and tempo, the more likely the statement is to be received most completely by the listener. A demand is merely an affirmative statement declaring unequivocal terms to another party.

DESIRE

Desire is a manifestation of the ego, not the soul. Desire, like ego, focuses upon (so-called) future benefit. Desire is not focused in the present moment. If someone is focused in the present moment, they feel no lack, for they feel completely cared for by the universe, as their every need is perfectly provided for — and thereby feel no desire. The soul is always focused in the present moment. The soul never experiences desire.

The person who experiences desire is not present as they are fixated on a future outcome. So, desire blocks presence. Without presence, the person cannot see truth. They do not clearly see the true nature that resides beneath the surface of any experience. Truth is seen only when present — not when focused upon so-called future (or so-called past).

Desire withers the heart (energetic heart chakra and, thereafter, physical heart organ). This occurs as disappointment associated with unrequited desire leads to frustration, which is an expression of core anger. Anger is a powerful emotion, represented by the element fire. Of course, fire is capable of great devastation in an instant. Anger is equally powerful. Anger, symbolized by the element of fire — obviously the most virulent of the elements — when not released in an appropriate manner is buried, and eventually attacks the core aspect of the energetic template. In a sense, frustration (anger) is a precursor to depression. Depression results from cumulative anger turned inward over time. The early phase of unrequited desire is characterized by the classic Taoist symptoms of impatience and intolerance. This represents an energetically *closed* heart chakra. Without desire, we are at peace, satisfied with whatever the moment presents — and thereby not apt to focus upon the so-called future.

The Buddha's teachings focus, in large part, upon how to transcend desire.

DISCIPLINE

I consider myself a typical product of western culture. I grew up in a suburb. I now reside in a city. I am somewhat educated. As a youth I toyed with competitive athletics and music. Regardless of the task I sought to master, I was taught that discipline was, at least, a semi-weekly practice and, at best, a daily practice. I was taught that (discontinuous) discipline, spanning a few hours per day, five days per week, at most, was adequate preparation and training for most tangible activities — such as relative *mastery* of sports, music and even academics. Certainly Western training (academics, sports, music, etc.) did not advocate discipline as a *moment-to-moment, continual* process.

Discipline, in simplest terms, is simply listening to, and heeding, the inner voice (of right action) **in every moment.**

I was fortunate to have access to the homes of three great beings,
one a Tibetan lama (Arjia Rinpoche),
one a Taoist teacher (Bruce "Kumar" Frantzis),
one a Hindu guru (anonymous).
Each man maintained a constant
moment-to-moment
discipline.
This never faltered.
This is true discipline.

In ancient cultures, mastery of self, personal evolution, was taught as a constant, moment-to-moment practice. This may sound like a radical standard of performance — but such discipline accelerated one's evolution. Why? Because, in the words of Dr. Jack Miller (formerly affiliated with Loyola University, Chicago, Illinois), *"Psyche requires rhythm for growth."* In other words, the subconscious mind and core energetic template respond positively to repetition. The greater the repetition, the quicker and more complete the transformation. Continual repetition, in every moment, brings most efficient and profound positive change.

To the best of my understanding, gained through observation, I noticed Tibetan lama Arjia Rinpoche's constant discipline of asking himself, in every waking moment, "What is right action?" And now in this moment. And now in this moment. Ad infinitum. What was equally powerful was that Arjia Rinpoche presumably would then listen to whatever his inner voice silently stated was *right action* and would actually *DO* whatever his inner voice said to do. Unlike most beings he would not ignore his inner voice's suggestion.

The practice of right action, in every moment, becomes easier over time, given repetitive practice; one begins to notice that life flows more smoothly when listening to, and heeding the wisdom of the inner voice.

To the best of my understanding, through observation, it seemed that Bruce "Kumar" Frantzis would practice abdominal breathing in every moment. This is a simple yet difficult practice. Simple in that abdominal breathing is a no-brainer exercise that takes five seconds to learn. Difficult in that it takes great discipline to maintain abdominal breathing with every breath (as the monkeymind dislikes this practice). Note that abdominal breathing becomes easier with practice and, after a while, becomes more comfortable than profane (shallow, a.k.a. "chest") breathing.

In summation, discipline is simply the practice of listening to, and doing, whatever the inner voice (of right action) decrees *in every moment*. For further explanation, see the section *Action – Right Action*. In brief, right action is any activity that best supports the good of all beings (in every moment). See the section on *Breath* for an expanded explanation of abdominal breathing.

EMOTION

Humans are holistic beings. We are comprised of a bodymind with a surrounding and permeating energetic aura. The components of the bodymind, body and mind, so intimately communicate with one another that they are best considered as a single unit. Body and mind communicate with one another through a variety of mechanisms including the nervous system and endocrine system.

Emotion is the body's response to thought. Emotion is entwined with the workings of the endocrine (hormonal) system. For instance, suppose a stimulus occurs in the external environment: a tornado off in the distance. The *thought* of a tornado and possible circumstances triggers brainwaves. This thought, in turn, influences the endocrine glands (pineal gland, thyroid gland, hypothalamus, etc.) to secrete hormonal messengers into the bloodstream—in this specific example to warn the body that it may need to take, in this specific case, *fight or flight*. Specific hormones then attach to specific internal organs (and other cells) that correspond to the specific thought pattern.

In essence, *hormones transcribe thought, located in the brain, into emotion, located in the body* (specifically in the internal organs). In this way, anger is *bioenergetically* stored (resides) in the liver; fear resides in the kidneys; worry resides in the spleen, pancreas, and stomach; and sadness and sorrow reside in the lungs. In the case of seeing a tornado, we likely experience a pre-cursor thought of fear, which transcribes as the emotion of fear, which is biochemically/ bioenergetically expressed in the kidneys.

Emotions are an essential and natural aspect of human experience. Feeling emotion is appropriate and healthy. Burying or denying the feeling of emotion is inappropriate and eventually may lead to compromised physical health. Why? Because emotion is bioener-getically processed and held in the body. Healthy flow of emotion through the body—a cycle of feeling, then releasing (*in an appropriate manner*) any given emotion, supports physical health. But, in contrast, feeling emotion but then burying—rather than releasing—emotion creates a pool of *stuck* (stagnant) emotional energy in the body, which ultimately may catalyze physical dysfunction and/or physical disease. Thus, we must learn to process and release emotion efficiently and effectively. This process accelerates self-awareness/ evolution.

> *The mind holds only questions.*
> *The body holds only answers.*

Emotional intelligence is tantamount to *wisdom.* Emotional intelligence is simply mentally-based intelligence integrated into the body— through experience. True intelligence is holistic in nature (i.e., rooted in the bodymind unit) —whereas mental intelligence is not integrated (into the bodily aspect of the bodymind). The body is a direct conduit to the wisdom and energy of the Tao (i.e., Heaven and Earth).

Thus the body is said to hold truth and, thereby, "only answers." This contrasts with the mind that isn't plugged-in to the complete holistic (bodymind) circuit and so holds questions but not true answers (as truth, in the highest sense, is attained by accessing the wisdom of the Tao and Heaven and Earth).

EMOTIONAL REACTIVITY

It is appropriate to remain *non-reactive* (yet, paradoxically, not un-feeling) at all times, regardless whether faced with *positive* or *negative* outcome. Note that the ego (mundane — *lower vibration* — aspect of the personality) judges situations as *good* or *bad*. In contrast, the soul (or *higher* aspect of personality) does not judge situations as good or bad but, rather, understands that all experiences are helpful to our evolution, as we learn from all experiences. The egoic aspect of the personality is *reactive* — in response to its judgment of experiences as good or bad. The soul *experiences,* yet does not *react* — as it does not judge experiences (again, as good or bad). *It is natural and essential to feel emotion — as emotion is an integral aspect of the (body-centered) human experience.* [See the section entitled *Emotion.*] *Yet it is neither natural nor essential to (inwardly or outwardly) react.*

As we evolve — i.e., process information less from the perspective of ego and more from the perspective of soul — we become ever-more *lovingly non-attached* to (and so less judgmental of) situational outcomes — as more and more we reflect and express the nature of the soul (which is non-reactive). Such compassionate detachment allows us to view situations from a more objective perspective. The objective viewer remains detached from emotional reactivity. The objective person releases emotion from the body in an appropriate manner (see *Emotional Release*), and cognitively realizes there is nothing to lose (as all experiences are a win-win opportunity — as we learn from all situations), which serves to minimize emotional reactivity. *The objective person feels (pure) emotion, yet is free from (disproportionate) emotional reaction.*

As a radical example, let's consider the Taoist perspective of how the Buddha might *react* to extreme circumstances. For example, how would the Buddha react if his car was stopped at a red light and the driver of a car behind him had a bad-hair day, and so was constantly honking at the Buddha's car? How would the typical human react (after a long, challenging day at the office)? Whereas we might yell an expletive or two out the window, or make a hand gesture toward the person honking, or perhaps simply feel a bit of anger without outward expression, the Buddha's reaction would be predictably consistent and simple. *He would feel the immediate surge of emotion* (in this case, perhaps anger, if appropriate), *but would **immediately** release the emotion.* Since the emotion had already released *from his body,* no residual (*stagnant,* that is, *unhealthy*) emotional energy remained in his body to serve as kindling for emotional reactivity.

We, on the other hand, would likely feel an immediate surge of anger (and/or other emotions), hold the anger in the body—without immediate release (unless we had learned emotional release techniques through Qi Gong or related training), and this energy would surge, causing us to expel the energy through an inappropriate—i.e., *reactive*—manner, such as extreme outward expression (yelling, flipping the honker off), while concurrently inwardly storing the cumulative stagnant emotional energy. The greater the amount of emotional energy held inside, the greater the likelihood of an eventual reaction (i.e., *going postal* on someone). The process of emotional release is explained in the following section.

EMOTIONAL RELEASE

The master walks a fine line.
She allows herself to feel pure emotion (in the body)
yet paradoxically
immediately releases emotion (from the body).

The highly-evolved individual fully experiences pure emotion. And instantaneously releases emotion from her energetic field. Why is this essential? Why is it necessary (*healthy*) to feel emotion?

Recall that we are a holistic unit, a unified bodymind. And recall that emotion is the body's response to thought. So, if we are not feeling emotion, we are not integrating our thoughts into an emotional form in the body (internal organs and, arguably, all cells), and so we are not connected to the bodily aspect of self. To be whole (i.e., fully integrated, a complete energetic circuit), we must experience the body, i.e., feel emotion.

Yet, paradoxically, *whereas it is essential to health to feel emotion fully, we must resolve emotion ASAP, since unresolved emotion accumulates in the subconscious core, promoting eventual physical, mental, and additional emotional dysfunction and disease.*

So, what does it mean to *resolve* emotion?

Again, recall that *thought* is bioenergetically *stored* in the mind, whereas *emotion* is bioenergetically stored in the body. To resolve *unresolved* (i.e., unhealthy) thought patterns, we eventually learn through trial-and-error experience (typically inefficient) to read or receive instruction from another (teacher, psychologist, etc.) in order to understand eventually the *unhealthy* thought pattern. We can then consciously choose to engage in a healthier pattern of thought.

> *Reveal*
> *Re-Feel*
> *Release*

To resolve emotion, we must release the emotion from the body. How?

To resolve (i.e., heal) emotion:

1) We must first *reveal* (dig up previously-experienced emotion that prior we were not ready to deal with and so buried in the subconscious mind);

2) We must again experience (i.e., feel) the emotion that prior we buried. We must *fully* feel or, more aptly, *re-feel* the emotion—with the hope that this time around, we are ready to process and release the emotion appropriately, rather than shove it under the rug. We must not run away from the feeling. We must engage the feeling (a.k.a. emotion) completely. Only then may we completely release the emotion.

3) *We may then release the emotion.* How? By engaging in activity centered in the physical senses (optimally while feeling real-time emotion)—i.e., through creativity (expression through the five senses) and through reception of stimuli through the five senses. [See *Voice of the Soul: A Call to Action* for a more detailed explanation.]

An example: to release unresolved thought and emotion triggered by a nearby tornado, we must A) release fear-based thought from the mind, and B) release the emotion of fear from the body (specifically, from the kidneys).

To release fearful *thoughts*, we may read a book or speak to an expert regarding tornado behavior, in order to gain cognitive understanding of how to survive such a storm and, in theory, no longer hold fear-based thoughts if another storm approaches (as we would learn how to safely deal with the storm).

And, to release fear most efficiently—this emotion of fear being stored in the kidneys in response to fear-based thought—we may engage in non-action while feeling real-time emotion. To do this, we express through the five senses (*while feeling fear*—this is the key!)— initially through vigorous (cardio-based) movement. Then express through whatever sense was most developed as a child (i.e., did you lose track of time more so when moving—via dancing and sports— via creation of visual art, or via creation of music?). Again, this must be engaged (activated) while feeling real-time emotion. Such activity, in and of itself without feeling real-time emotion, is not *psychemotionally* cathartic.

As a specific example, to release emotion, I initially move vigorously (workout) while feeling an unresolved emotion; then I create music— play guitar—while feeling the emotion. Then I may write and sing lyrics regarding the unresolved emotion, while playing guitar again, while feeling of the emotion—to honor and release the emotion.

Note: in all cases, first move the body! And drink a liter or two of water. Why? Emotions are water-soluble (and so dissolve in the water we drink and release), and movement causes the internal organs— where unresolved emotions are stored—to move, which catalyzes release of emotion from the internal organs. Further, since expression through the five senses (*while feeling real-time emotion*) serves to affect the subconscious energetic template directly, movement—again, along with creation (of visual art, music)—serves to cleanse the subconscious template of unresolved emotion. Receiving body-based stimulation, again, while feeling real-time emotion—(massage, body-work, etc.), sound (CDs, concerts), visual stimulation (color, geometric patterns, beautiful vistas such as sunrise and sunset), aromatic stimulation (aromatherapy), and taste-related stimulation (food, spices, etc.)—serves to help release unresolved emotion from the subconscious template (and Antahkarana). [See *Voice of the Soul: A Call to Action* for further explanation of emotional release.]

There is a protocol (i.e., an appropriate sequence) to efficient and effective release of emotion. To heal most efficiently, we initially release the greatest density of trauma (stagnant energy) from the body, followed by release of progressively subtle stagnant energies (from body, mind and surrounding energy field).

EMOTIONAL RELEASE PROTOCOL

To release unresolved emotion (specifically, emotive-psychenergy) and physical manifestations of dysfunction efficiently, initially dance or run/swim/bike/walk while feeling the emotion. Ideally, raise the heart rate for at least twenty minutes (or what will not overtax your body). Then create based upon the emotion (art, music—especially if innately "wired" as a visual artist or musician at birth). Thereafter (or possibly concurrently), initiate cognitive healing—by reading relevant explanatory books or through professional consultation to help the cognitive mind to recognize and take responsibility for recurring patterns of mental beliefs that introduce negativity into the bodymind (and Universe).

EMPATHY

Empathy is the ability to stand in another's shoes
and truly understand their circumstance
as perceived through their senses.

It is impossible to empathize when engaged in the ego (egoic aspect of personality). We must engage our soul (and unconditional love) when attempting to perceive another's perspective of the circumstances they face.

46

Empathy versus Compassion. *Empathy differs from compassion in that compassion is the ability to recognize that another person has a beautiful soul — and to engage them as that beautiful, flawless soul — thereby forgiving (yet appropriately dealing with) the flawed aspects of their personality. Empathy, on the other hand, involves the ability to feel what the other being feels — from the aspects of their personality.*

Whereas it seems that empathy should be relatively effortless if Person #1 has experienced a situation similar to that experienced by Person #2 — this is not so. Why? Because Person #2's perception of the identical experience will likely differ from Person #1's perspective. Thus empathy is challenging — as one must literally sense the perspective of the other, as seen through *their* five senses (eyes, ears, nose, mouth and physical sensitivity).

Paradoxically, we must *feel emotion completely* to release emotion completely. Allow emotion to flow fully through you to the core of your being, for as long as needed, to completely experience *pure* emotion. Then release the emotion.

EMPTINESS

It is the space within
not the exterior shell
that defines the value
of a vessel.

Paradoxically, emptiness is the mother of creation. Yet, creation resolves into emptiness. This cycle of creation-emptiness illustrates the impermanence of the dualistic world. For instance, the empty space of the womb gives birth to the infant. The infant ages and, eventually, the physical body disintegrates, reverting back to (physical) emptiness.

Emptiness of ego
Fullness of soul

Similarly, it is the emptiness of the mind that gives birth to higher understanding — via fullness (presence) of soul — connectedness of the soul to the Tao (i.e., Heaven and Earth). It is said that the master's mind is like that of a child (or idiot). She does not think. As though a conduit from the Stream of Consciousness, she allows the flow of inspired thought to move through her. She does not create evolved thought. She is a conduit for conscious information sourced by the infinite wisdom of Heaven and Earth. By emptying the mind of all thoughts (loving detachment), she is able to access highest consciousness and thereby receive inspired information.

How do we achieve emptiness? Through non-action. [See the section entitled *Action – Non-Action*.]

ENERGY

Prior to the invention of the electron microscope, energy was *visible* (via the third-eye energy center) only to *"sensitives"* – adepts skilled in attainment of a state of profound meditation. Of course, everything is comprised of energy. Ancient people didn't feel the need to understand the technical aspect of phenomena as Western scientists do today; if something existed, it existed – regardless whether the Ancients would explain why. They took things at face value. They accepted that energy exists, without understanding its exact nature. The wise people of that era, who sensed energy (through profound stillness meditation), were revered for their insight. Energy was described as light. Nothing more. Nothing less. In contrast, today's quantum physicists label aspects of energy in terms of sub-atomic particles – which are, effectively, tantamount to light. The ancients knew that the *essence* of energy is light. And, the ancients realized that energy (light in its many forms) demonstrates specific traits. They recognized that the energy of the body inspires blood flow. In other words, acupuncturists observe that "blood follows chi." And, subsequently, blood inspires physical health. Additionally, they discovered that energy follows intention. Whatever we intend manifests in the physical realm (subject to certain factors such as whether an outcome is aligned with the truth of who we are at the core – i.e., our life purpose and life service, and whether aligned with the lessons we are meant to learn – i.e., karma).

ENERGYWORK

Energywork is facilitation of energy movement through a person's energetic field (auric field including physical, mental and emotional aspects of the bodymind).

Traditional Chinese Medicine prescribes a hierarchy of healing described by a progressively-subtle protocol that includes acupuncture, herbal medicine, and qi gong (energywork without props).

Methods of self-performed (so-called "self-help") energywork include, but most certainly are not limited to, T'ai Chi, Qi Gong, Yoga, etc. Methods of energywork performed for the benefit of another person include, but are not limited to, Acupuncture, Qi Gong therapy, Reiki, Chi Nei Tsang, Jin Shin Do, Craniosacral Therapy, Trager, etc.

EVOLUTION AND ENLIGHTENMENT

Enlightenment
is each and every moment.

It is not something to attain
in the so-called future.
It is something to be
now,
in this moment,
and this moment.

Regardless how un-evolved members of the human race may seem, each of us is destined ultimately to attain enlightenment (a highly evolved state of being succinctly described as heightened self-awareness). How is this possible?

We are on Earth to *learn*. This is the purpose of our existence. Sorry if you were hoping for something a bit more glamorous! The process of learning affects us to the core. As we learn, we literally transform the very shape of the (subconscious and conscious) energetic template that defines who we are (our level of evolution — i.e. our level of self-awareness). In objective terms, evolution is measured by the strength and purity of our inner energetic template. The inner template may be described by an acupuncturist as the Central Channel—a mostly vertical energetic cord reaching infinitely upward (to Heaven) and downward (to the center of Earth). The strength and clarity of this channel (specifically known as the *Antahkarana*) are measured by the width and verticality of this energy cord. [See *Antahkarana*.]

> *The Antahkarana bisects the precise center of each of the major seven chakras. The wider and more vertical the Antahkarana, the greater one's evolution. The Antahkarana of an enlightened being is wide and vertical, free of horizontally-skewed kinks.*

In contrast, the mortal being's Antahkarana (approximate Central Channel) is kinked at numerous locations. In other words, there are horizontal skews defacing the vertical integrity of the Central Channel. These kinks map where we have not yet resolved fundamental life lessons. As we gain mastery of life lessons, we straighten the kinks of the Antahkarana—eventually bringing verticality to its entire length (and thereafter widening its breadth)— the objective definition (i.e., measure) of enlightenment.

> We attract polar (*both-ends-of-the-spectrum*) experiences to help us resolve the dualistic nature of reactivity by the egoic aspect of the personality when faced with life situations; our eventual mastery of these life lessons serves to straighten the kinks in the Antahkarana. Again, the kinks are unaligned aspects of our being, which represent ego-alignment rather than soul-alignment, regarding specific life issues.

> The ego's reactivity swings like a pendulum. It attracts trial-and-error lessons in the form of polarized experiences— which, again, eventually serve to straighten the Central Channel (the objective energetic measure of our evolution). For example, you might date a guy/gal with certain traits and subsequently date another guy/gal with (superficially) opposite traits. Each experience teaches lessons that help us to resolve relational issues.

* *

THE *BHAGAVAD GITA* ON
EVOLUTION AND ENLIGHTENMENT

The *Bhagavad Gita,* one of the most profound books of East Indian (Hindu) wisdom, describes—through a conversation between a person (Arjuna) and the Infinite (The Beloved)—how to "worship" in the highest manner both during life and at the time of death, suggesting that such practice supports our evolution.

The Beloved explains that our being is the essence of all things—i.e., we are connected to everything. Our actions affect everything. Our creative power is limitless. During every moment we are alive, truest worship is simply being present—maintaining all focus upon the present moment. And *at the time of death, whatever we focus upon shall dictate the journey of the soul.* Thus, at all times we must fight to remain present. We must resist the doubt and negativity of the monkeymind (which seeks certainty—a condition which is non-existent in the dualistic, material world; as the only certainty is the Infinite). If you are strong enough to maintain focus on the present moment you will innately learn highest truth—via the whispers of truth shared by the vehicles of the inner voice—namely, intuition, dreams and synchronicity. The monkeymind cannot access truth—as it cannot access the present moment (as ego can focus only upon so-called past or so-called future). Only the soul can access the present moment— and convey its wisdom via the inner voice.

Presence—tantamount to transcendence of the monkeymind—is supported by the practice of body-centered consciously-aligned activity (such as yoga, t'ai chi and meditation). Presence is supported by non-action. [See the sections *Action: Non-Action* and *Meditation – Stillness Meditation.*]

Maintain presence via soul-aligned activity [see Volume 2 of *Anatomy of the Human Fabric* Trilogy, *Voice of the Soul: A Call to Action*] during every waking breath. Then, at the time of death, draw the breath up between the eyebrows—to the third-eye chakra, and you will connect with the Beloved (i.e., experience moments of blissful presence – otherwise known as enlightenment—in which you will experience joyous peace, feel full of vitality, feel a heart filled with love, and feel no desire whatsoever for material attachments—true *emptiness*). In sum, all focus is upon the feeling of a heart filled with love, with breath centered between the eyebrows, and a mind focused upon the Beloved and nothing else. All this, while uttering "Om."

Given such practice at the time of death, you may transcend the karmic wheel, no longer needing to experience cycles of pain and suffering (if aligned with the state of your karma).

Note: balanced meditation requires focus not only on the Third-Eye energy center (between the eyebrows) but equally upon the Lower Tan Tien energy center (two to three inches beneath the navel); focus on the Lower Tan Tien, especially using abdominal breathing (see the sections entitled *Breath* and *Grounding*) inspires innate grounding.

EXPRESSION

When thoughts regarding a topic are clear, express yourself completely, then remain outwardly silent, and let go of the thought internally. If thoughts are unclear, practice non-action (soul-aligned activity) to open mental and emotional flow. When thoughts are clear, express completely, remain silent, then let go of the thought internally. [See *Voice of the Soul: A Call to Action* for a detailed description of soul-aligned activity.]

If a party does not clearly receive your expression, you may consider restating the essence of the communiqué. If they again cannot comprehend the statement, or refuse to listen, do not try to force your point upon them. Accept the miscommunication as a temporary condition. Consider trying to make the point at a later date. If the individual then does not fully receive the information expressed, exercise discernment regarding the root cause of the miscommunication. Is the other party simply exercising resistance to you? Does the other party disagree with your perspective and so refuses to hear your point? Are you not communicating effectively — i.e., are you not using terminology or concepts that are readily understood by the other party? As a rule of thumb, take full responsibility for the miscommunication. Do not blame the other party (or yourself). *Look at how you contributed to the miscommunication.* And, if the other party is merely resistant to you, examine your discernment (i.e., re-consider why you choose to communicate with this individual at all). Recall that people are in our lives for a reason, a season, or a lifetime. Examine the lesson taught by miscommunication—as there is a lesson to be learned.

EXTREME CONDITIONS

All conditions are favorable.

The Meditation Master Who Prefers to Remain Nameless

In the extreme situation, or extreme end of a range of variation, yin transforms to yang, and yang transforms to yin. Such radical transformation is witnessed during healing crises. This is a blessing. We draw healing crises to ourselves when we otherwise do not choose to heal. In other words, we subconsciously draw progressively challenging and uncomfortable situations (i.e., progressively extreme conditions) to ourselves for the express purpose of motivating ourselves to shift (repetitive) unhealthy beliefs and unhealthy conduct. We become so uncomfortable that we are no longer able to tolerate existing conditions—so, at long last, we are inspired to change unhealthy patterns that block our health, happiness and evolution. In essence, we are forced to our perceived *breaking point* to inspire us to shift the way we think and react, to bolster healthy thought patterns and minimize emotional *reactivity*. So, all conditions are favorable, since all experience presents an opportunity to learn and evolve.

FAILURE

Failure is a paradox. On one hand, there is no such thing as failure (or *mistakes*)—as long as we choose to learn from prior misguided experiences (i.e., so-called *mistakes*). The soul does not recognize any activities as *failed*, again, as long as we choose to learn from the experience. Yet, on the other hand, the egoic aspect of the personality (monkeymind) tends to falsely label misguided activities as mistakes, and concurrently points a finger of blame (either outwardly or inwardly).

The soul does not judge. The soul sees the big picture. The soul realizes that foolhardy activities serve as an opportunity to learn. Failure exists only if we refuse (i.e., are not ready) to learn from the consequences of prior misguided activity.

FAITH

The Tao abhors a vacuum.

Anonymous

What is the meaning of the statement "*The Tao (a.k.a. universal wisdom) abhors a vacuum?*" Recall that the reason we exist is to learn. How do we learn? Through experience. How do we experience? We are presented appropriate props of experience — namely, people, objects and events (which trigger us to re-feel previously buried emotions) — so we can resolve previously unresolved lessons. So, the concept of faith is quite straightforward. Faith simply means that we trust that the Tao will (always) present the appropriate props (people, objects and events) that will help us learn (i.e., evolve). Having faith in the Tao means we believe the Tao will provide what we need to evolve — no matter what circumstances may be. Always. Note that patience is the ultimate test of faith. Conversely, patience is effortless when we hold faith.

FAMILY

Great gifts await those who choose to maintain close contact with family (except where instances of abuse or overt callousness are evident). Family members are among the most efficient catalysts of personal growth (through relational dynamics of mirroring, projection and transference). [See sections regarding *Mirroring, Projection* and *Transference.*] Many lessons are learned and mastered through interaction with family. Biological family lineage shares genetic disposition. Biological and non-biological family (adopted family) share similar environmentally-instilled patterns of mental and emotional reactivity. Family members not atypically share intimate (non-sexual) and sustained communication and history. These factors create ripe terrain for interpersonal dynamics that readily trigger mirroring, projection and transference — dynamics that support personal transformation (as eventually we release emotional reactivity). Additionally, the entwined nature of familial relationships is also the spawning ground for understanding of trust.

You were born into a *specific* biological or adopted family *for a reason*. Like any relationship, a family member may be in your life for "a reason, a season or a lifetime." Esoteric Eastern philosophers propose that we subconsciously select our parents, and even siblings, pre-birth. They believe that we choose parents and siblings through whom we shall learn and master specific unresolved fundamental life lessons.

Your biological family is not necessarily your (so-called) *spiritual family*. The phrase "spiritual family" infers a kindred community of like-minded and like-hearted people. Since we select family members who serve as triggers for unresolved lessons, we may or may not *resonate* (i.e., feel mental, emotional and/or spiritual compatibility) with that person. This is obvious in families where abuse occurs. The abuser is not an aligned partner, yet is a trigger of learning (whether the lesson is discernment — to distance oneself immediately from the trigger, or whether the lesson is eventual resolution with the abusive party — only after the abuser has profoundly shifted their conduct, words, and intention).

FEAR (THE GREAT ILLUSION)

Fear (except fear of actual imminent physical harm — which activates bodily fight or flight response) is based upon illusion. Thereby, some philosophers say that fear is not real. And yet, paradoxically, the body responds to the illusion of fearful thought as though fear is very real. So, to the body, fear is real. Recall that emotion is the body's response to thought. And that the bioenergetic imprints of the emotions are stored in the internal organs. Specifically, the body stores a bioenergetic imprint of fear in the kidneys. Fear has an adverse effect upon the kidneys. The most direct way to protect the kidneys (and body) from physical transcription of fearful thought is to see through fear. By setting all focus upon *faith*. See fear for what it is, mere illusion, and you will always be safe.

Fight or flight bodily response is appropriate at times, when physical survival is threatened. Fear of physical harm may be described as *real*, whereas mental, emotional, and spiritual fear are illusory.

Once fear attacks the kidneys, it is imperative to release the bioenergetic impact from these precious internal organs. To do so, see the section entitled *Emotional Release*. [Also see *Voice of the Soul: A Call to Action*.]

A barometer of fear is the inverse of the strength of one's faith. Compromised faith promotes fear. A heightened sense of faith diminishes fear.

FOCUS

> *What we focus upon*
> *in any moment*
> *is all that we are.*

Ancient Taoists believed that all that exists is this moment. And this moment. And this moment. Ad infinitum. Further, they believed that all we focus upon in any given moment is all that we are. For example, if we focus upon love, in this moment, all we are is love. And we radiate the vibration of love to the world.

All we are is what we choose to focus upon in any given moment. We focus upon the outer world via the five senses (taste, smell, vision, hearing, and tactile sense), the mental aspect of the bodymind, and the emotional aspect of the bodymind. If we focus upon creativity, we are creativity. If we focus upon positive mentality, we are positivity. If we focus upon emotion, all we are is that specific emotion. And we radiate that emotion throughout the universe.

Focusing upon core creativity (and body-centered breathing) while experiencing real-time emotion helps us to be *present* (mindful of, i.e., focused upon, the present moment). When focused upon the present moment, we are aligned with the soul—and guided by the wisdom of Heaven and Earth—via the soul.

FORGIVENESS

To err is human.
To forgive
is to tap immortality
in the moment.

Forgiveness requires us to recognize the humanness in ourselves and, thereby, others. We cannot completely forgive another unless we learn to forgive ourselves. To forgive ourselves, we must deal with both the cognitive (mental) and bodily (emotional and bioenergetic) aspects of the bodymind.

To forgive someone, we cleanse mind and body of *resentment* toward that person. Resentment consists primarily of anger (of subtle and not-so-subtle degree). We resent the actions, words and/or thoughts that contradict our preferences. We are angry that—what we perceive to be—adverse conditions have been placed upon us, conditions that we do not prefer. So, at some level, regardless how subtle, we feel anger toward the person.

How do we forgive a person?

To forgive another in complete fashion, release negativity from **both** body and mind. The cognitive mind must (mentally) acknowledge the human-ness of the other party—through a combination of empathy (putting oneself in another's shoes) and compassion (loving respect for all living things). The process of cognitive forgiveness is accelerated by release of anger, sadness/sorrow, fear, and worry, from the physical body (from the liver, lungs, kidneys and spleen/ stomach/pancreas, respectively). To release emotion, see the section entitled Emotional Release.

To mentally recognize (understand) the human-ness of another, we must first understand our own human-ness. We must cognitively acknowledge our own mortality. Our weaknesses. Our indiscretions. Our misguided thoughts, words, and actions.

To forgive a person, must we trust or like the person? The answer is a resolute *no.* Nonetheless, the process of forgiveness is favorable — as we release anger from the bodymind. A companion to the lesson of forgiveness is the lesson of discernment. If we do our best to evolve — i.e., to gain mastery of ourselves — and if the other person does not, or, worse yet, if the person remains in a regressed emotional and mental disarray of irresponsibility, it may be appropriate to distance oneself from the other person. For example, if a person is physically abused by another, unless the other person undergoes extensive and pro-found therapeutic counseling and sustained transformation, it is likely best to avoid the person (until the person gains a modicum of self-awareness — although this might not occur in this lifetime).

That we are forgiven and forgive does not indicate that it's okay to continue to err. To the contrary, when we are forgiven by another, we must take complete responsibility for the indiscretion we created, and address the unresolved aspect of our conscious and subconscious minds that caused the indiscretion. When forgiven by another, if we can sincerely apologize while focused upon the present moment, (exercising empathy and compassion for the harmed party), and take full responsibility for our indiscretion, we most efficiently release the unresolved aspect of ourselves.

To forgive we exercise pure compassion and empathy. [See sections regarding *Compassion* and *Empathy*.]

FORM — BEYOND FORM IS ESSENCE

Beyond (technical) intelligence
is sublime understanding

Form is outward (superficial) expression of essence. Our physical, mental, emotional, and spiritual form is a precise mirror reflection of our inner energetic template. Nothing more. Nothing less. Form in the material plane is created (magnetically attracted and thereby developed) by our core energetic template (subconscious and conscious mind). Whatever we believe in any given moment manifests outwardly at a subtle level (if aligned with karmic lessons we need to resolve). Any sustained belief pattern of sufficient intensity and duration, whether *negative* or *positive*, manifests in physical form. [See the section on *Timing*.]

Essence is everything (from the perspective of the soul) yet nothing (from the perspective of the egoic monkeymind).

FULLNESS

Paradoxically, it is the capacity of the empty space within, not the surrounding shell, which bestows the value of a vessel. Similarly, it is the capacity for emptiness of the mind, which bestows connection to Heaven and Earth (fullness). Fullness (of the bodymind/soul) seems empty (to the egoic mind). We feel full when connected to the soul and body. We are a complete circuit when tapping the energy of the soul and body. And in this state of consciousness, when connected to truth, we innately recognize connection to the infinite—fullness of heart/soul that is tantamount to emptiness of (lower) mind (i.e., transcending the monkeymind). Presence renders fullness of soul— as the soul is connected to the Tao. For this reason, Buddhist "emptiness" refers to emptiness of ego, fullness of soul (i.e., connection to the Tao via the present moment).

GOODNESS

True goodness welcomes both saints and sinners. True goodness does not distinguish whether the receiver of goodness *deserves* its call. Thus, true goodness is tantamount to grace—love given yet unearned. Or, arguably, earned by the very birthright of being alive.

All deserve goodness—regardless of prior indiscretion.

Forgiveness is a form of true goodness—wherein love and light are given regardless of prior indiscretions.

NOTE

Namaste (and Jai Baghwan). These Sanskrit terms express the idea "my soul recognizes your soul." This is a tool through which to transcend judgment of the personality (and ego) of another being. This perspective facilitates the flow of goodness. These two are traditional greetings that proactively set the tone of any meeting.

(end of NOTE)

GRATITUDE

Gratitude is a necessary ingredient for present-moment focus and happiness. And, conversely, is a result of present-moment focus. Gratitude is open-hearted surrender to the reality of the present moment. Gratitude is acceptance of all aspects of the present moment: acceptance of the conduct of people, outcome of events, etc. Gratitude lives in the present moment. Gratitude blooms from the soul. Gratitude does not focus on the so-called future. Nor does gratitude focus upon the so-called past. Gratitude is the perspective of the soul. Ego cannot focus upon the present moment. Ego focuses only upon the so-called future and past. The ego knows no gratitude. Ego always wants more, more, more — and so precludes happiness. Buddhist tradition emphasizes that we must be empty of ego to be present. So, to be grateful, we must be empty of ego.

GREATNESS — TRUE GREATNESS

True greatness can be achieved only if one does not reach for greatness. To seek to be perceived as great, by others, or even oneself, is an act of ego. To serve in the greatest way is an act of the soul. Even the most subtle activity may be great, if it serves the world and universe in right manner.

The Taoist view that all that exists is now and now and now (ad infinitum) reminds us that one may act in a great way in one moment, yet not in the next moment. Thus, true greatness is a discipline, an ongoing internal commitment to right action in *every* moment.

True greatness may be perceived by the ego as weakness, foolishness, stupidity and/or inaction. Yet it is precisely the opposite. For example, the greatest general knows that it may be suicide to take the first move in battle. It is wiser to initially retreat a bit, than to force a situation without understanding one's opponent. To the ego this may appear as weakness.

GROUNDING

When reaching for the stars, we, at times, may lose our footing. To avoid losing connection to the core self, the body, and the Earth, stay present (focused upon the present moment, be mindful) via a practice of non-action. [See *Action — Non-Action.*] Rooted in present-moment consciousness, we are no longer randomly affected like a leaf in the wind. Focused upon so-called future (and past), we lose connection to the Earth — and ourselves. Centered in the present moment, we become genuine.

The family that practices mindfulness flourishes. A country grounded in the present moment is a world leader, an example to the rest of the world.

Technically, in energetic terms, the bodymind is described as *grounded* (rooted) when the bodymind's Central Channel (a.k.a. Antahkarana — a meridian of energy that flows from Heaven down through the precise center of each chakra, down to the Earth, and back up in an eternal cycle) connects to the Earth (Earth Center or Earth Star) via the feet (which send energy downward through the heels of the feet, and receive upward flowing energy from the Earth through the balls of the feet). To achieve this state, it may be helpful — while meditating — not simply to focus on the third-eye (chakra) located between the eyebrows, but additionally (or primarily) to focus upon the Lower Tan Tien, located two to three inches below the navel. This focusing upon the Lower Tan Tien will enhance grounding via strengthened connection to Earth (while concurrently accessing Universal (Heaven) energy. Note that meditation on the Lower Tan Tien primarily accesses Earth (grounding) energy, and secondarily taps Heaven energy. Focus on the Third-Eye chakra primarily accesses Heaven energy and, secondarily, connects to Earth (grounding) energy.

Andrew R. Sadock

HEALING

We are holistic beings. In other words, we consist of a mind and body that are so intimately entwined that we, most aptly described, have a *bodymind*. The bodymind consists of physical, emotional, intellectual, and spiritual components. Each of these aspects of the human fabric is comprised of energy. Note that since these aspects are interconnected they may not be viewed as though in a vacuum. In other words, *we completely heal any aspect of our being by considering all other aspects of our being*. More specifically, we heal all body or mind conditions by treating both body AND mind — not by treating body or mind alone.

Traditional Chinese Medicine views health in terms of flow of energy (primarily through twelve internal organ-related energy meridians). Meridians are rivers of energy that flow throughout the body. Like a healthy river, a healthy bodymind experiences open flow of energy. Dysfunction and disease, like an unhealthy (mucky) river, are caused by blockages of flow.

We may *directly* heal our physical aspect (physical symptoms — but typically not the cause of the symptoms) by employing Western (allopathic) medicine — including physical medicine (via MDs and allopathic practitioners).

We may *directly* heal our physical aspect through Eastern (holistic) medicine including acupuncture, herbs, ayurvedic medicine, homeo-pathy, bodywork, diet, etc. In my experience, I have observed that *allopathic medicine is necessary in cases of potentially lethal, acute illness (wherein death is imminent within 24 hours without proper treatment)*. For example, surgery is required if an appendix bursts. The alternative is death. In case of exceptionally severe systemic infection, again wherein death is imminent without immediate treatment, antibiotics are mandatory (via intravenous induction).

But, in cases where death is not a probable outcome, then alternative holistic medicine methods are worth trying. Why? Holistic medicine is most effective for chronic illness — due to absence of side-effects. Additionally, holistic medicine is typically much less expensive than allopathic medical procedures and medications. Unlike allopathic methods, which treat only one aspect of the bodymind, holistic

62

methods support integrated (concurrent) healing of physical, mental, emotional, and spiritual aspects of the bodymind. Finally, holistic methods, unlike allopathic medical methods, do not simply mask symptoms — as holistic methods actually heal every level of the body-mind, helping to heal the core cause of the dysfunction/disease. For example, consistent yoga and/or t'ai chi (qi gong) practice may effectively treat physical chronic illness, unaligned patterns of thought, emotional stagnancy, and spiritual misalignment. Ingestion of herbs may support healing of all levels of dysfunction. Acupuncture may support healing of all levels of dysfunction.

We may *directly* heal our emotional (and psychological) aspect via allopathic psychiatry and psychology; and/or via holistic psychology qi gong therapy, yogic therapy (for example, Phoenix Rising), and other modalities. Yet other healing methods may *indirectly* support healing of our emotional aspect — diet, herbs, aromatherapy, spices, energywork, bodywork, and other holistic healing modalities.

The hierarchy of healing in Traditional Chinese Medicine (TCM) consists of acupuncture (bottom rung), herbal medicine (middle rung) and qi gong (energetic medicine comprised of intentional breathwork and movement, highest rung). Each modality may be used concurrently to heal physical, emotional, intellectual and spiritual aspects — again, as all aspects of our being are inter-connected.

HEALING — ENERGY MEDICINE

Energy medicine (a.k.a. vibrational medicine) may be employed to heal all aspects of our being (physical, emotional, intellectual, and spiritual aspects). Everything is made of energy. So, all our aspects consist of energy — including areas of dysfunction and disease, which are simply energy blockages. We may effectively treat energetic deficiencies and blockages using energetic medicine (vibrational medicine). Chinese qi gong, East Indian yoga, Japanese Reiki, and a multitude of healing modalities may be employed to heal all aspects of our being.

However, be wary of energy healers — as the profession is under-regulated. Use your intuition — if a holistic healing professional seems professional and *feels right*, employ their services. If a healer doesn't seem professional or feel right, walk away after the initial interview. Trust your gut feeling (intuition). And, if intuition approves, then call references, etc. — do your homework to confirm that the healer is appropriate for the service you seek.

HEAVEN AND EARTH

Heaven and Earth are entwined. They represent polar energies that vitalize and balance the bodymind (including auric field). A light bulb cannot light unless it is connected to both positive and negative polarities. The bulb will not light if connected solely to either positive or negative polarities. Thus, positive and negative (polarities) are of equal value. In the dualistic world, positive and negative create one another — for without one there cannot be the other (as their very existence, is based upon their relativistic dynamic).

Taoism and other ancient philosophies infer that the goal of life is to become a conduit of the energy (wisdom) of both Heaven and Earth. This is tantamount to surrender of the personal will to universal (collective) will. This is supported by personal transformation. Conversely, an effective barometer of one's personal evolution is one's ability to access the pure (unfiltered) voice of the wisdom of Heaven and Earth.

Technically, *as we evolve, the primary (core) energy meridian* (the Central Channel or Antahkarana, an antenna-like, vertical energetic channel that leads from Heaven to Earth — and vice-versa — through the precise center of each chakra) *gains width and verticality.* It widens and becomes straighter in a vertical direction and substantially widens in breadth. It becomes a greater vertical river. The theory is that the wider and straighter (more vertical) the Central Channel, the greater the influx of wisdom (energy) of Heaven and Earth into the bodymind — such that we become progressively stronger *conduits* of such wisdom. In essence, we innately gain highest-quality wisdom via the Central Channel's connection to Heaven and Earth. The monkeymind contains, at best, (cognitive and abstract) *knowledge*. Knowledge transcends to *wisdom* only when transcribed into the body by (hands-on) experience, which transcribes the mind's knowledge to the cells of the bodily aspect of the bodymind. A holistic definition of wisdom is cognitive or abstract knowledge (held in the mind) that is expressed through experience to all cells of the body. The quality of information held by the monkey-mind pales in comparison to the quality of wisdom contained in Heaven and Earth. By becoming energetically open (a.k.a. a conduit) to the wisdom of Heaven and Earth, we actually access MUCH higher-quality information that has a direct impact upon the quality of your life (and evolution). [See sections entitled *Antahkarana* and *Chakra* for more detail.]

Paradoxically, due to existence in the dualistic material world, Heaven and Earth cannot exist without one another. They are relative concepts. Yet, each carries unique energy to the bodymind.

The wisdom and energy carried from Heaven to the bodymind is of highest vibration, and radiates (primarily) through the upper chakras. This universal energy nurtures and supports the possibility of infinite loving, artistic and telepathic ability.

The wisdom and energy of Earth, as presented to the bodymind, carries grounding to our energetic circuits, which *completes the circuit* for full awareness. Rootedness to the Earth supports emotional release, balance and self-awareness. Connection to Earth is supported by an intention of mental focus upon body-centered breathing (especially Abdominal Breathing, a type of breathwork featured in Qi Gong, Yoga, and other philosophies), which brings the energy of the breath to the Lower Tan T'ien (an energy center located 2 to 3 inches below the navel).

HOPE

Hope is as illusory as fear. Both arise from the egoic, thinking self (monkeymind, rather than from the body and soul). Like fear, hope is an illusion. It is not real. Fear is merely a perceived lack of love (i.e., lack of light). Similarly, hope is not grounded in reality.

How do we resolve this paradox — that hope is not real and yet seems essential? The answer is straightforward. Simply, hope — like fear — is a perception of the ego, not soul. Again, both are illusory. Hope merely focuses upon materialism (tangible and intangible) that will at best satisfy the desire of the ego (but does not support evolution of the soul).

In contrast, faith, unlike hope, is a perception of the soul. Faith is real. Faith is the understanding that the Tao will present you with everything you need, precisely when you need it (to support your soul's evolution). **Don't hope. It's an empty practice. Rather, hold faith.**

HUMILITY

She who tries to impress, does not. She who tries to sparkle in the eyes of others instead casts a shadow. In contrast, she who does not assertively exhibit herself allows others the opportunity to see her light. The Master does not aggressively radiate her Light externally, for the purpose to impress. Rather, the Master allows flow, and surrenders to the great Tao, the nameless, benevolent, creative, universal energetic force (consciousness). Thus, the Master is sculpted by the Tao, rather than self-guided and self-defined by the ego. This is humility.

She, who does not know that she is great, is truly great. Why is this? She does not judge herself. She is not in judgment. She, thereby, is not focused upon ego. Thereby she is focused upon soul. Recall that what we focus upon in any moment is all that we are. Soul-focus requires pure humility. Soul-focus accesses truth. Thus it is great.

Humility is the eternal practice of the Master. Why? The Master dedicates her every thought to focus upon the soul. *Humility is surrender of the ego.*

Note that I did not say that humility is *surrender BY the ego* — as the ego never surrenders. The ego is defeated by conscious mental focus upon the soul (via soul-aligned activity). [See *Voice of the Soul: A Call to Action.*] *We surrender the ego by focusing upon soul — through disciplined exercise of soul-aligned activity.*

Only given genuine humility and great effort may we profoundly shift (i.e. evolve, transcend) from a relatively unevolved subconscious energetic posture to an enhanced internal energetic vibratory state.

IDENTITY (PRIMAL)

To know one's core primal identity, we must travel to the core. To do so, we must go beyond the reach of the physical senses. We must blunt the mind's cleverness and intellect. We must unravel all emotional knots. We must soften our glare to a vision of surrender rather than that of seeking. We must settle our dust until underlying essence is innately revealed — through willingness, surrender and, most significantly, grace.

True identity is simply accessed. Focus every moment upon the Tao. Unite with the Tao in every moment. This is your true identity — found only when focused on the present moment (soul alignment). Unification with the Tao — simply by being present — illuminates your uniqueness — your unique life purpose and life service. [See section entitled *Action – Non-Action*, and Volume 2 of *Anatomy of the Human Fabric Trilogy*, entitled *Voice of the Soul: A Call to Action*.]

IMBALANCE

Quite simply, to counter imbalance, focus upon balance. Center subconscious and conscious energies by practicing soul-aligned activity (non-action). Focus upon the soul. Stay centered in the Tao (universal force). See the section entitled *Non-Action.*

IMPERFECTION

The world cannot be improved upon in its essence. It is sacred. A great paradox is that the world's imperfection is perfect. Imperfections are perfect as they trigger us to evolve. Without imperfection we could not grow.

IMPERSONALITY

To understand impersonality, we must first define *personality*. Personality is the aspect of self that holds freewill. In each moment, personality chooses to focus upon either soul or ego (the default position). Personality, as defined loosely, consists of both mental and emotional aspects. The mentality of personality is derived from *thinking*, a function of the mind. The *emotionality* component of personality is derived from *feeling*, a function of the body. Recall that emotion is the body's response to thought. We must feel. Feeling emotion is a sign that we are connected to our bodily aspect. Not to feel emotion is to be numb to life, unaware of the body, which is tantamount to disconnection from the self.

Does impersonality, as alluded to in the *Tao Te Ching*, infer a state of minimized emotionality? Yes and no. Yes—as the outward manifestation of emotions/feeling seems non-existent. No—as inward experience of emotions is *complete*. Impersonality, simply stated, involves efficient and complete processing of emotion—*without inner or outward emotional reactivity*. Note that a propensity to *react* infers that aspects of the personality are unresolved (i.e., unevolved)—and thus are subject to bursts of spontaneous reactivity when triggered by people or events. To be fully alive and aware, we must feel. Completely. Yet, when resolved (i.e., evolved), we need not be outwardly reactive. The Master feels and immediately releases thought and emotion—without outward reaction. This is impersonality—or, more aptly stated, transcendence beyond personality.

Impersonality infers lack of outward emotional reactivity—yet complete and efficient (inner) processing of emotion. In other words, the self-aware individual feels pure emotion and *immediately releases it* from the bodily aspect of the bodymind. No residual unresolved emotion remains in the body, so the person is not *triggered* to outwardly react (in defensive or offensive fashion).

Impersonality is objective—as impersonality reflects the perception of the soul—whereas the soul is an objective observer. Thus, impersonality does not subjectively interpret life's situations. As the *Tao Te Ching* states, impersonality understands the personal (i.e., is aware of the emotionality and mentality of the individual), yet knows not to focus on subjective interpretation and experience.

Impersonality may easily be misinterpreted as non-caring. But this could not be further from truth. Impersonality objectively accepts the world as it is, and thereby acts in the highest, most loving way, in all moments. Without subjective reactivity (of the personality/ego), impersonality is able to view situations objectively, to deliberate objectively, and to pose solutions objectively that promote the highest good for all parties to any transaction (including all inhabitants of planet Earth).

Esoteric, ancient philosophers believed that we must transcend emotion to achieve objective (pure) mentality. What does this mean? Are they saying that we must not feel—i.e., must not experience emotion? No. Again, to the contrary, we must learn how to feel (pure) emotion completely—in the moment. And then learn how to release the emotion completely—preferably as soon thereafter as possible (notably, in a best-case scenario it is possible to experience and release emotion in the same moment). As an analogy, consider any given point in a healthy river—water flows in, yet flows out, at the same time.

Summary: Paradoxically, to the outer world, impersonality may appear as *non-feeling* (non-emotionality). Yet, in actuality, impersonality is an experience of pure emotionality (and efficient and complete release of emotion). Complete processing of emotion, with complete emotional release, allows freedom from subjective misinterpretation of situations and people—by dissolving emotional *cloudiness* that otherwise arises in the (unresolved) emotional aspect of the bodymind, which blocks clear vision and perspective.

INSTITUTIONS

It is essential that institutions are aware of where they fit in the big picture. A conscious institution clearly understands precisely what it contributes to society. It is aware of this boundary. It does not overstep its appropriate boundary. It respects the role of other institutions. It does not seek to compete with other institutions, rather, it seeks to synergize and synchronize with other institutions.

INTELLIGENCE

Awareness is knowledge and understanding of all aspects of one's self. Intelligence is knowledge of others and external situations and conditions.

The Hierarchy of Intelligence

[Highest]

Intuitive Reasoning Centered in the Soul
Integrated Reasoning Centered in the Bodymind
Cognitive and Abstract Reasoning Centered in the (Lower) Mind

[Lowest]

Intelligence exists in many energetic forms. *Cognitive* (mental) *understanding* (loosely defined as "knowledge") involves that aspect of mentality located in the brain. This is superseded by *integrated understanding* (loosely defined as "wisdom": cognitive understanding that through experience—particularly through kinesthetic experience, through experience centered in the other four physical senses, and through emotional experience—gains energetic grounding in the bodily aspect of the bodymind).

Note that wisdom is knowledge that has been integrated into the bodily aspect of the bodymind via hands-on experience. This is energetically superseded by *intuitive reasoning*, intuitive intelligence). Intuitive intelligence is sourced (i.e., accessed) by the soul, not by the monkeymind. Intelligence sourced by soul is accessed via dreams, intuition (gut feel), synchronicity, and miracles.

The mind holds only questions.
The body holds only answers.

This adage suggests that lower mind accesses limited information and that the bodily aspect of the bodymind, home to emotion and connection to soul, accesses enhanced information that is sourced from the Tao (i.e., Heaven and Earth).

70

INTUITION

Intuition is *gut feeling*. Sometimes intuition is as subtle as the quietest whisper, and passes in an instant. At other times, it's as loud as a jackhammer and persistent. Intuition is the voice of the soul. The soul speaks via four mechanisms. Internally, the soul speaks to us via dreams and intuition. Externally the soul speaks to us via synchronicity. The soul carries universal truth to us via dreams, intuition, and synchronicity. In contrast, the mind (specifically, the monkey-mind or the profane/mundane mind) presents mundane information. The soul taps the Stream of Consciousness, an immortal, infinite information flow that transcends linear time and space.

Ancient philosophies believe that soul-borne information may power mortal beings to transcend mortal performance. Thus, the wisest artist allows her intuition to guide her. The prudent scientist remains free of concepts, and allows her mind to stay open to the voice of intuition.

There is no substitute for intuition. Cognitive understanding (mind-centered thought) cannot supplant the immortal wisdom provided by intuition. Recall that cognitive (brain-centered) thought is labeled as *knowledge*. Body-centered (integrated) thought/learning is labeled as *wisdom*. Intuition transcends both mortal knowledge and wisdom. When the body's intelligence recedes, brain-centered thought may step forward (as cleverness) — but cleverness is not a substitute for integrated learning. Similarly, if we are not connected to soul, knowledge and wisdom cannot fill the gap of forfeited eternal information.

KARMA

What goes around comes around.

Anonymous

We come to the physical plane for the purpose of mastering fundamental and progressively advanced life lessons. Initially we learn and master basic lessons (of relatively high density -- e.g., don't murder, rape, steal, covet, etc.). As we progress, we learn and master lessons of progressively subtle density (e.g., humility, patience, compassion, simplicity, letting go, etc.). This leads to self-awareness, pragmatically yet simply defined as understanding one's life purpose (core creativity) and life service (to help the world). Life's lessons are the means to our ultimate end—namely self-awareness (a.k.a. consciousness, ascension, enlightenment, self-awareness, etc.). The goal of the soul as it travels on its journey is to align all aspects of who we are with Heaven and Earth—so that we may become conduits (living examples and mouthpieces) of consciousness.

To learn, we encounter lessons that trigger unresolved wounds that we previously buried deep within the core of the subconscious mind (as we were not then ready to resolve the psychenergetic/emotional wound). Recall that *to heal we must again reveal (i.e., feel)* feelings that prior we weren't ready to resolve—i.e., feelings that were buried long ago (or not-so-long ago) in the recesses of the subconscious mind.

Karma is appropriation of natural order (justice) based upon cause-and-effect. Although frequently misinterpreted as punishment, karma's lessons are anything but that. Rather, karmic lessons simply intend to teach. Karmic lessons are gentle or not-so-gentle experiences that force us to learn appropriate (right) activity for life situations. Where prior we acted, spoke, or thought in an inappropriate manner, karmic lessons teach us to approach a similar situation in a new (i.e., appropriate) way. Suppose you choose to treat *Person A* in an inappropriate manner—perhaps by ignoring their opinion when they speak. A karmic lesson might present a scenario in which *Person B* subsequently ignores your opinion—so you can feel what *Person A* felt when you ignored their opinion. Via *Person B's* action of ignoring your opinion—a simple and efficient mechanism—you would gain empathy for *Person A's* feelings, and learn not to treat people in that way.

Karma is directly linked to the subconscious mind. What is the subconscious mind? The subconscious mind is the womb of instinct—prehistoric tendencies regarding survival of the species, involuntary function, and unresolved thought and emotion—unresolved thoughts and emotions that we buried beneath the surface, as they were too uncomfortable to resolve at the time. Through karmic mechanisms, the conscious and subconscious aspects of self attract people, objects and events that help us to act, speak and think differently than we did before—via the magnetization of the karmic wheel of cause-and-effect. Theory states that the subconscious mind may energetically attract approximately eighty percent (obviously a rough guestimate) of our material world experience—to induce natural order (justice) via karmic balance.

LABELS (MATERIAL IDENTIFICATION)

Labels are impermanent,
limiting,
counter-productive,
for without labels
people innately do what is right
as they are happier.

Labels are counter-productive. They are grounded in judgment. They are predicated upon, and enhance, separation—which is illusory, as in reality everything is connected. Labels are limiting. The ego attaches to labels as they promote a sense of (false) certainty. A false identity. Labels describe you as *this.* And me as *that.* Yet you are not *this.* You simply are. In each moment we shift. We simply are what we are in each moment (as, arguably, we are precisely what we focus upon in any given moment). Labels give the ego a sense of material attachment that promotes a false sense of security. Without such security, the ego, the restless monkeymind, squirms to find certainty—an illusory concept. The ego is always focused upon the so-called past and future—neither of which is real. Recall that the so-called past is unreliable as it is merely one's perception of what happened. And the so-called future is obviously unreliable as it is speculation. The only certainties are change, the Absolute (the Tao), and the present moment. Ego cannot focus upon the present moment. Only soul can focus upon this moment. And this moment. And this moment. Ad infinitum. Since ego is constantly looking to create a sense of certainty in the so-called future (which isn't real), material identification helps placate the ego. Yet, identification with any aspect of the material realm is impermanent, for this is the true nature of the dualistic, material universe. The ego seeks certainty in every moment. Labels give the ego the solace it seeks, for a moment or two. Until ego perceives that the labeled object or event no longer comfortably fits and so no longer gives the ego energy (as ego is a vampire), and ego again searches for its next *fix* like a junky.

A dualistic society judges based upon labels. Without labels, it is difficult to judge another. Judgment is the lowest form of vibration. Judgment stems from ego. Ego feels better when it compares itself to another and perceives itself as superior. This is not the nature of truth. Truth simply is. Truth is incomparable.

The lesson: Just do the right thing and let things take care of themselves. Do not label — as labeling is tantamount to judgment.

False societal labels and institutional infrastructure serve to limit the flow of a country. The more a country or organization labels, and thereby compartmentalizes its components, the more difficult to navigate in an efficient and effective manner.

LEADERSHIP

The best leader guides so effectively that followers believe they led themselves. Her hand is perceived as invisible. She proactively creates effective systems that quietly guide.

Effective leadership is quiet. It empties people's minds (egoic monkeyminds) and fills their hearts and souls (with heart-felt purpose — not egoic ambition). The best leader follows the will of the people; thereby the people do not know they have been guided. The best leader serves as an example and does not exert their personal will. Leadership is like frying a fish: too much poking ruins either. The world appreciates a great leader.

The second-best leader is loved by the people. The third-best leader is respected. The second-worst leader is feared. The worst leader is despised. [See the section on *Confusion*.]

LEARNING

Why are we born? Why do we exist? Simply, *to learn*. To master fundamental and increasingly subtle life lessons. We are born imperfect so we can rise above imperfection and, in the process, learn (i.e., evolve). And in many cases, also learn how to help others to transcend situations similar to those we once faced. All that we may take with us from this lifetime is what we learn during our days on Earth. What we learn is all we get. Sorry if you were expecting something a bit more glamorous.

There is a hierarchy of learning. We are holistic beings comprised of body, mind and soul. Cognitive learning, centered in mind, is the lowest form of learning. Mind collects knowledge. Integration of mental knowledge into the body creates bodymind-centered wisdom. We may transcend mind and body — culminating in learning aligned with the soul, which is rooted in intuition. Higher learning is bodily integration, rather than mental compilation. Highest learning is accessed via intuitive reasoning, centered in the soul,

LETTING GO

A paradox ...
Why do we focus on accomplishment and accumulation
of people, things, and information
for the initial forty-plus years of life?
For the soul purpose of learning how to let go —
for one cannot learn how to let go
without initial attachment.

To let something go, completely, we must first allow it to flourish. Why is this? For unless something runs its full course, we may miss lessons that we were destined to learn in the relationship or dynamic. If all lessons are not learned, or at least triggered (i.e., initiated wherein the seed of the lesson is planted), a relationship is not essentially resolved. In youth (and through the initial thirty-five years of living) we focus our energy upon accomplishment and mastery of material activities. In other words, we increasingly attach to materiality — people, objects, information and events. Then, at approximately age thirty-five, we gradually begin to learn how to let go. Of people. Of things. Of desired events. Of (ego-based) hopes (but not of soul-aligned *faith*). Of (ego-based) dreams. Until eventually **we learn how to let go gracefully, with intimate understanding of the impermanent nature of all things, thus understanding that we are merely letting go of impermanence.** In effect, we lose nothing — as materiality is an illusion. Letting go teaches us the challenging lesson of *loving detachment,* and reveals truth regarding impermanence.

> *Nothing is impossible*
> *because she has let go.*
> *In the place of ultimate surrender*
> *[of personal will]*
> *anything is attainable*
> *[if aligned with universal guidance].*

Steven Mitchell, *Tao Te Ching*

LIBERATION (FROM KARMA)

Liberation from karma occurs at the conclusion of the cycle of karma. In theory, this occurs once an individual has mastered life's fundamental and subtle lessons. How long does this take? It varies for each of us. Each of us will achieve liberation (a.k.a. self-awareness, enlightenment, ascension). Some quicker than others. In theory it takes many lifetimes to attain complete self-awareness. In each successive lifetime, we consciously and subconsciously strive to gain mastery of lessons passed unresolved from prior lifetimes. Some lessons may be quick to learn and master. Other lessons may take lifetimes to master. Liberation occurs once an individual masters life's lessons. In theory, once this occurs the person no longer continues on the karmic wheel. In other words, the person no longer needs to experience additional lifetimes since they have learned all fundamental life lessons. They are liberated from the wheel of karma.

LIFETIMES — PRIOR LIFETIMES

What creates the unique traits of infants? Is it simply genetics?

Western science argues that genetics creates the predisposition, the seed that if watered by an environment of experience, given certain supportive parameters, will sprout certain traits. Yet, how do we explain Mozart—the child prodigy who at age four was writing compositions that were nothing less than the work of genius? Was this simply a foreseeable yet unlikely genetic probability positioned at the extreme end of a statistical bell curve? Or was this the result of a process greater than Darwinian genetics? Could it be that Mozart's obvious gift, especially as exhibited at such a tender age, was merely an extension of musical mastery attained in prior lifetimes (one or perhaps many) that he was somehow able to recall consciously?

In support, let us ponder why we have such large brains — yet consciously tap only ten percent (an estimate) of the capacity of the cerebral cortex? Could it be that the other ninety per cent of the capacity of the cerebral cortex stores information, perhaps from prior lifetimes (and/or taps into information from etheric data sources, such as the Collective Conscious)?

The purpose of our existence is to learn. We are on Earth to master fundamental and subtle life lessons. How do we learn? Through experience. What are the props of experience? People, objects, and events. We experience dynamics with people, objects, and events to trigger and learn fundamental and progressively advanced lessons.

However, we can learn only so much in one lifetime, as we can only experience so much in one lifetime. Therefore, to master the many lessons that life throws at us, Eastern philosophers proposed that we live many lifetimes. Certain lessons may take longer than other lessons to master. Some lessons may take many lifetimes to master. Some lessons may be mastered in a single lifetime.

One theory says that we learn one major lesson per chakra per lifetime, and many minor lessons per chakra per lifetime. As a great anonymous Hindu meditator said — "Who knows?"

LIGHT

True to form, the *Tao Te Ching, speaking in paradox,* states that the path to Light seems dark. What does this mean? To evolve, we must completely heal. To heal, we must again feel what we were not ready to feel in days, years, and lifetimes past. We must transcend the shadow component of the mind to experience Light. Why? Unfortunately, the best analogy I can present is tantamount to *zit theory*. A pimple heals only by releasing the toxins beneath the surface. We heal the emotions in similar fashion. To heal emotion, we must reveal (i.e., RE-FEEL) emotion similar to that previously buried in the subconscious mind. It is not enough to think about an emotion. Then, while feeling the emotion, we release the emotion using appropriate tools. [See the book entitled *Voice of the Soul: A Call to Action*.] Thus, the path to Light seems dark, as we must re-experience *dark* (unresolved) emotions to release them, then move forward to Light. *The path forward, circles back* (to heal). To become complete we must empty ourselves (of emotional and energetic stagnancy).

The experience of Shakti, the opening of the Third-Eye chakra, located between the brows of the forehead, in the center of the cranium, accesses infinite Light (a.k.a. the *Divine* Light). This experience has been reported through the millennia by meditators. Some individuals who have experienced near-death experiences also report seeing light, without opening their eyes. In theory, light contains unlimited information. Therefore, the experience of Shakti accesses infinite information. In this manner, through profound meditation, the *Tao Te Ching* states that the master "does everything by doing nothing" — i.e., the master, through meditation (which appears to be doing nothing from a superficial perspective) does everything (as she connects to infinite information). Again, be aware that the *Tao Te Ching* speaks in paradox and, at times, a bit tongue in cheek!

LINEAGE (FAMILY SYSTEMS)

The following discussion may seem utterly esoteric, yet it is of substantial practical value. Many Ancient and contemporary cultures believe that we live many lifetimes. They state that the soul continues on its journey even after the gates of physical life close. The soul lives eternally, *dropping the body* at the conclusion of each lifetime as it continues on its path toward self-awareness. As discussed previously in this text, some esoteric ancient philosophies theorize that preceding reincarnation the soul considers the lessons it intends to master in the coming lifetime. In so doing it selects parents whose life paths (and lessons) are consistent with its intended path — i.e., the soul chooses parents who will present situations that contain lessons that the soul needs to learn.

The incoming soul may choose parents with whom it has prior familiarity—perhaps they were friends, siblings, parents, children, employees, employers, etc. of the soul in prior lifetimes. Or the soul may choose parents with whom it has no prior history. Either way, the dynamic between the parents and child (incoming soul) will trigger unresolved lessons for each party to the dynamic. For instance, the incoming soul (child-to-be) may choose parents who are likely to abandon or otherwise mistreat the child if this lesson is in the best interest of the evolution of the souls of parents and child— perhaps, if for no reason, than to balance the karmic scorecard (in the hypothetical case that the child-to-be had abandoned or mistreated others in a prior life).

Some ancient and contemporary cultures believe that we maintain an energetic connection when those before us (parents, grandparents, great grandparents, etc.), after us (children), or lateral to us (siblings) in the family chain pass on to the next plane. And that the familial chain of beings, and in the extreme, the chain of all beings, remains connected energetically (as truly we are all connected; note that boundaries of linear space and time do not exist between any two beings—this is illusion.).

Ancient theory suggests that we chose our parents (and indirectly siblings, grandparents, and preceding generations) for the purpose of resolving our internal unresolved energies through lessons that our (omniscient) souls foresaw before conception, as these *specific* beings, given their unresolved internal energy patterns, would most efficiently and effectively trigger the life lessons our souls need to master. Similarly, our parents chose their parents for the same reason—to be triggered to evolve.

Ancient esotericists believed that it is not merely the parents (we would say, the DNA) that carry the basis of the familial bond, but also that something more ethereal, as though strands of energetic thread carry unresolved lessons of one generation to the next generation. In other words, *lessons that are not learned by a former generation pass to the latter generation*, which must learn and master the lessons that were not mastered by the generation before. The theory states that once the latter generation resolves the lesson, the resolved energy flows back to the (souls of the) prior generation, resolving the energy of the prior generation. Sorry if this esoteric theory sounds a bit *distant!*

The Ancients believed that *as we play out our karmas and life lessons, the resolution of these energies heals not just us, but all in our familial lineage*— all those before (and those following us, as the so-called past and so-called future are accessed through the present moment). In theory, the principle of *connected lineal healing* purportedly has a noticeable effect over five generations in either direction. Hence, any emotional and psychenergetic healing that you experience benefits not only you, but five generations of family ahead and behind you in the family chain. Again, I apologize if this sounds a bit *out there!*

This principle takes place even where one is estranged from their biological parents—as the bio-parents still benefit from whatever healing is accomplished by their progeny. And, should one have adopted or spiritual parents, they too benefit from one's work. As does the entire human race and all within the Universe, although less directly. *As you do your work, your family chain is benefited.*

LOVE— SELF-LOVE (VERSUS SELFISHNESS)

Paradoxically, we must take care of ourselves to care for others. We can fully give to others only if we fully love ourselves. Self-love benefits all others, in each moment. Yet selfishness benefits no one. Self-love feeds one's soul (in a manner aligned with one's highest truth). Self-love supports one's highest path of evolution at the level of the soul. Since all souls are connected, self-love feeds all souls. Selfishness, feeding one's ego, benefits no one. Selfishness tends to the desires of the ego—and nothing more.

LOVE—TRUE LOVE (LOVING NON-ATTACHMENT)

True love may seem *indifferent.* Why? True love is unconditional. True love supports another on their highest (soul-aligned) path regardless what form the path may take. True love is selfless yet complete, infinitely giving yet fully able to receive. True love supports another even where their path may be juxtaposed to one's personal desires.

True love acts. False love talks. True love embraces the imperfections of another as dearly as their attractive qualities. True love is detached. It allows another to be who they truly are. It inspires another to travel wherever appropriate. It is eternal. It is infinite. It does not own. Nor does it possess. Rather, it inspires, nurtures, and cares.

MANIFESTATION

Careful what you ask for
as you just might receive exactly that.

The process of manifestation occurs from the inside out. Our innermost intention creates our material reality. The *Tao Te Ching* states that being is born of non-being. In other words, materiality blossoms from the soup of the infinite, which is sculpted by our etheric, conscious thoughts and, more so, by our innermost subconscious state of energy (theory states that the subconscious template magnetically attracts 80 per cent of our external experience, to help us to evolve — i.e., heal unresolved, subconscious issues).

We influence materiality through two mechanisms. First, through direct action. Direct action is activity that focuses upon a specific material (tangible or intangible) outcome. An example of direct action is making a telephone call to a person we wish to speak with. Second, we may influence materiality non-directly, through non-action. Non-action is activity that focuses upon raising our inner energy levels (vibration). As our inner vibration is raised, we naturally attract people, objects and events of relatively higher vibration (who carry needed lessons to us). [See *Attraction — The Law of Attraction*, above.]

When manifesting through direct action, there exists the danger that we may manifest what our ego, rather than soul, desires — which likely will not be best for us at a soul level, in the long-run.

MANIFESTATION — RIGHT MANIFESTATION

To assure we manifest what is best for us, employ non-action. Non-action calls upon natural order (aligned with our soul, accessing the infinite wisdom of Heaven and Earth) to raise our inner vibration. The soul knows what is best for us in the long-run; our limited mind does not. Thus, it's best to initiate the process of manifestation by first engaging in non-direct activity (non-action), followed by direct action once the right path is visible and obvious.

MANIFESTATION — A FIVE-STEP METHOD

A five-step system facilitates manifestation — but only where the intended outcome is aligned with one's highest path. Simply stated, the method follows:

1) State your preferred result using as many words as necessary to convey all aspects thereof [completed by: *"with the intention of being of highest service to the Universe"*].

2) Pray for the result — but only when your energy is grounded (connected electromagnetically to the energy of the Earth). [See the section entitled *Prayer.*]

3) Refine your objective using as few words as possible.

4) Optional: Before sending it up to the Universe, command that any negative, confused energies underlying your intention be returned to you. You may feel any impurities return to you at this time. You may experience sensation in the chakras (especially chakras one through three). You may release these energies from your energy field by using breath and intention (the essence of qi gong).

5) Send the thought-form up to the Universe. Visualize the thought-form leaving your body as a white balloon rising above.

This method is very powerful, especially when used on a repetitive basis. This method encourages manifestation from wholeness, bringing lessons of greatest and highest value. Note that in theory manifestation by an enlightened being is immediate. The second a thought arises, physical manifestation of that thought occurs. This *power* is earned by those who have learned to control their thoughts and energies in every moment. Enlightened beings, such as the

Buddha, focus only upon positivity. Their intention is unconditionally loving in every moment. They intend and manifest only outcomes that support the highest good of everyone. They have previously mastered the lesson of patience (the ultimate test of faith) and thus need not *wait* for any result. In contrast, note that we mortal beings wait for outcomes — as we are meant to learn the lessons of patience and faith. [See sections entitled *Patience* and *Faith*.]

MANTRA

See the section entitled *Sacred Geometry*.

MEDITATION – EYE MEDITATION

Eye meditation is a powerful means of communication which, in theory, transcends the communicative capacity of verbal words. Eyes are *windows to the Universe*. Sensitive beings can sense who someone is by looking into their eyes. We feel their essence. And we can feel their connection to the higher realm: highest consciousness. *The practice of eye meditation helps us connect to this highest power through focus upon another's eyes. During this exercise, we meditate, while looking intently into another's eyes.* Try it. You will find this to be a powerful experience. The longer you remain connected to the energy of higher power and the other person, the better. Employ this practice only with someone whom you trust.

MEDITATION – STILLNESS MEDITATION

> *All that we do is a precursor to stillness …*
> *Stillness is a paradox:*
> *silent, motionless,*
> *yet the most dynamic*
> *powerful state of being.*

Stillness is the optimal state of being. The most subtle state of being. The most powerful state of being. The most dynamic state of being. And the most natural state of being.

Andrew R. Sadock

Simple in theory.
Challenging in practice.

Stillness is the most powerful state of being. Why? Because when our center and being are still (vertically aligned), we become an antenna that is sensitive to the whispers of Heaven and Earth. Via the soul. We exponentially magnify our capacity to tap higher power, higher consciousness. We access subtle truth. We transcend the confines of linear space and time. We access our true nature. Our truth. Our life purpose. Our life service. The very reason for our existence. We smile inwardly. Simply by being still. When profoundly still, we access truth. We clearly hear the voice of the universe via the core voice within. Simple in theory; difficult in practice.

Meditation is
25 per cent willingness,
25 per cent surrender,
and 50 per cent grace.

The Meditation Master Who Prefers to Remain Nameless

How can we access stillness? By sitting still. By stilling all within. By stilling all our systems. *By transcending the senses, and the thoughts of the monkeymind.* How? By surrendering our personal will to universal will. Through the practice of humility. Humility is perhaps the most important ingredient—as we do not control meditation. **We do not meditate. We are meditated.** What does this mean? Our willingness to meditate causes us to assume the posture of meditation, sitting with back upright. Surrender means we allow higher power to move through us. We surrender ourselves to higher power. But humility, the key, is acknowledgement that a higher power is in control. We merely create the possibility for meditation. Grace meditates us.

Meditation is transcendence beyond the mind.

Specifically, to meditate, one method is to begin by moving the body (for ten minutes or more) such that your blood vigorously flows. This serves to help ground your energy in the body, influencing descent of energy from the monkeymind. Then, in a quiet room, or outdoors (best yet, sitting with a tree as a backrest), sit cross-legged or in lotus

84

position on the floor or ground, or in a chair with both feet placed firmly in front of you, with back vertically aligned. Breathe in through your nose and exhale through your nose or mouth, *focused all the while on the physical feeling of the natural rise and fall of the lower abdomen* (abdominal breathing) — the natural diaphragmatic expression of the breath in the lower torso. Energy follows focus (intention) and so continues to lower from the monkeymind into the body (lower torso energetic center, the Lower Tan T'ien). Maintain your attention on the rise and fall of the lower abdomen. Your focus may drift off. If distracting thoughts enter your mind, refocus your attention on the rise and fall of the lower abdomen. Initially meditate five minutes per day. After a week, increase meditation to ten minutes. When ready, increase meditation in five-minute increments. You need not follow the aforementioned instruction — as there are many ways to meditate, as described in a multitude of books, DVD's, and other media.

MEDITATION — WALKING MEDITATION

Walking meditation is a Buddhist practice. In walking meditation, we focus our attention upon subtle movements of the feet. Walking meditation helps ground the meditator. Grounding is literal energetic connection to the energy of the earth. By maintaining the mind's focus upon the feet, we lower our energy toward earth. This helps us access the energy and wisdom of the earth (and, secondarily, universal energy). A four-step walking meditation entails focus upon a heel raised a few inches above the Earth, gently touching earth, then (on the same foot) slowly lowering the ball of the foot to touch earth, then focus upon slowly lifting the heel (on the same foot), then focus upon the other heel raised a few inches above the Earth, etc. (and repeat the next three steps for the other foot). Practicing walking meditation each day.

MINDFULNESS (PRESENCE OF MIND)

Mindfulness simply means focusing one's mind (mental focus) upon the present moment. This is the essence of meditation. When our attention is focused upon the present moment, we access the soul.

When focused upon so-called past or future, we access ego. Presence and soul are brethren, as are so-called past/future and ego.

When present, we see all as new, as though we are a baby. We no longer take anything for granted. We do not presume to know anything. All situations are new. All moments are unique and precious. *We are infinitely connected and empowered.*

MIRROR(ING)

Our greatest nemesis is our greatest benefactor.

The person who triggers us to emotionally react most deeply (excluding cases of abuse) is our greatest teacher. What does this mean? The person who ticks us off the most, who hurts us the most, causes us to re-experience (re-feel) emotions deeply that we buried long ago in the recesses of the subconscious mind—as we were not then ready to appropriately process (and release) the emotions.

This is a gift, believe it or not, as it grants us another opportunity to heal (the unresolved emotions) … and evolve. Recall that *to heal, we must feel. Zit Theory* (sorry for the somewhat coarse analogy) states that the purulent exudates (pus) beneath a pimple must surface before the pimple can heal. This is tantamount to the analogy that to heal an emotion, we must feel the emotion (i.e., not merely *think* about the emotion). The emotion must rise from the subconscious mind into our consciousness, or we cannot heal the emotion. To cause the emotion to rise to the surface, we attract people, objects, and events that trigger us to re-feel previously buried emotion (i.e., cause us to feel anger, sadness, worry, etc.). These people, objects, and events are gifts—as they help us heal (even though, from the perspective of the monkeymind, the process may be less than comfortable).

A mirror is an individual whose (wounded) actions mimic our own (wounded) actions. *By observing the individual, we may remotely observe our wounded aspects.* For example, an angry person might attract another angry person into their lives—so they can see, feel, and otherwise experience their own anger as expressed by another being.

The following excerpt from *Conscious Relationship* offers a detailed explanation of mirroring, transference and projection.

The Mirror and Trigger. In accordance with the Law of Attraction, an individual shall invariably attract relationships that serve either to mirror or trigger their unresolved emotions. Why is this helpful? To heal (emotions), we must reveal and feel emotions buried deep in the subconscious aspect of the mind. *Relationship serves to dig up buried emotions — for the express purpose of helping us to heal, gain self-awareness, and evolve.* This is the reason for relationship. Two powerful healing mechanisms frequently occur in interpersonal dynamics — namely, mirroring and triggering.

Generally, mirroring occurs when an individual subconsciously recognizes patterns in another's behavior that mimic one's own unresolved patterns. For example, suppose Fred has not resolved the cardinal emotion of anger. Fred may learn how to process (emote, react, release) anger better by viewing Wilma as she *seethes* with anger. Wilma's over-reactivity with regard to anger mirrors Fred's own over-reactivity an unresolved anger. Wilma serves as a clear illustration (mirror) to Fred, which helps Fred to learn to cope with his own anger. Wilma mirrors Fred's anger. Wilma is described as a mirror (of Fred's unresolved subconscious behavior).

Generally, triggering involves one person's innate ability to activate a reaction in another person. For example, Barney may become reactive to a certain behavior by Betty. Betty triggers a response by Barney. Betty is described as a trigger (of Barney's unresolved subconscious behavior).

The mirror and trigger are healing mechanisms that help un-bury unresolved subconscious emotions. Again, to heal (and evolve) we must reveal (unbury and re-feel) emotion. There is no short-cut.

Relationship has been described through the millennia, and in numerous cultures, as one of the most powerful transformative tools available to help us evolve. Relationship is a magnifying glass — helping us to see who we truly are and, thanks to triggering (mirroring, projection and transference — described later), to evolve.

The Mirror — Theory. When Partner B's behavior mimics Partner A's unresolved behavioral patterns, Partner B serves as a mirror through which Partner A can see her own unresolved behavior. For example, Fred (Partner A) can see what his unresolved subconscious anger (or any emotion) *looks like* from a distance, when viewing the angry behavior of his wife Wilma's (Partner B). In effect, this affords Fred the opportunity to look in a mirror — to see his unresolved emotional reactivity clearly. Wilma's behavior serves as both mirror and magnifying glass through which Fred can view his own behavior, helping Fred to become aware of his unresolved emotional patterns that otherwise are hidden deep in the bowels of the subconscious aspect of monkeymind. Thus, this helps Fred to gain self-awareness and evolve. Presumably Wilma also gains from the relationship — through mirroring and triggering (and projection) provided by Fred.

An Example of Mirroring. Consider the case in which Fred has anger issues; his default reaction is hair-trigger anger. The mechanism of mirroring allows Fred to witness his own behavior. Whenever he sees Wilma become angry, he sees his own unresolved behavior (hair-trigger anger). She reflects his behavior back to him. He sees his own behavior as though reflected (and magnified) by his wife's actions. Hopefully, the observation of his wife's anger will help him to realize that his anger is inappropriate (and unhealthy). Perhaps this insight will inspire him to learn how to release the anger he carries buried in his subconscious mind.

The Trigger. Partner B serves as a *trigger* for Partner A's unresolved emotions when Partner B's behavior somehow causes Partner A to experience emotional discomfort, which is Partner A's feeling of the newly-surfaced unresolved emotions — which were previously buried deep in the subconscious mind. These newly-experienced emotions are brought to the surface by Partner A's perception of Partner B's behavior. To evolve, Partner A's previously hidden unresolved emotions must be revealed to be felt — and healed. Partner B's inadvertent triggering (unearthing) of Partner A's previously buried unresolved emotions serves to help Partner A to finally resolve these energies and, in so doing, gain self-awareness and evolve.

An Example of Triggering. Consider the case wherein Barney, who has repeatedly experienced prior bouts of the fear of abandonment, attracts Betty, who historically has experienced a repetitive pattern of the fear of engulfment (fear of intimacy). Betty's perceived need to run away when relational dynamics become *intimate* (emotionally intimate — not necessarily sexually intimate) consequently exacerbates Barney's fear of abandonment, while, concurrently, Barney's fear of abandonment triggers Betty's fear of intimacy (due to Barney's attempts to cling to Betty to preclude her from running away). The fears in each individual eventually are magnified to such extent that a condition is prompted in which either or both parties to the dynamics cannot escape these uncomfortable feelings — and thereby must initiate a legitimate healing process to resolve these unpleasant emotions and emotion-based thoughts. In this way, triggering promotes a healing crisis — which helps the triggered party resolve subconscious emotional/mental issues.

Projection (Pseudo-Mirror). In cases of projection, Partner A views the behavior of Partner B as a mirror of her own behavior — but unlike in the case of pure mirroring, inaccurately assumes that the intention underlying Partner B's action is identical to Partner A's intention — when engaged in similar patterns of behavior. In actuality, the action or words of Partner B may be created by an underlying intention that is dissimilar from that held by Partner A when Partner A is engaged in similar activity. This causes Partner A to project her underlying understanding onto the perceived image of Partner B's action.

So, projection, a pseudo-mirror, consists of two components. Mimicry of one's physical behavior (activity that mimics one's own activity), and the false assumption that when another person is engaged in mimicry, that their intention is identical — wherein it is not identical — such that the other person is engaged in similar activity but with divergent underlying intention.

An Example of Projection. For example, suppose that Desi and Lucy have dated for at least three months but are not yet committed to an exclusive relationship. Further, suppose that whenever Desi enters a bar that he fantasizes about meeting a *perfect* partner (who, of course, doesn't exist). Suppose that whenever Lucy enters a bar, she simply wants to meet friends — and does not fantasize about meeting a new partner. The result is that Desi, upon learning that Lucy plans to meet friends at a bar, may inappropriately suspect that Lucy will fantasize about meeting another partner when at the bar—inflaming insecurities within Desi. Unresolved issues buried deep in Desi's subconscious are dug up by Desi's worry about Lucy's intention (when in a bar)—as he has transferred his own intentions (to meet a perfect partner) onto Lucy's behavior (i.e., Desi believes that if Lucy enters a bar that she seeks the perfect mate, parallel to what he might be concerned with in similar situations. Even though Desi's assumption regarding Lucy's intention is incorrect, it is a pseudo-mirror of Desi's intention onto Lucy's actions, serving to reveal Desi's wounds. It thereby affords the opportunity for enhanced healing, self-awareness, and evolution (again—we must reveal and feel—to heal emotion). Desi is afforded the opportunity to see clearly what his underlying intention looks like from afar. This creates a disquieting experience for Desi and, thereby, serves as a platform for internal change and profound transformation.

MODERATION (THE MIDDLE WAY)

The polarities of the dualistic material world serve to teach us moderation. The pendulum of dualism swings to and fro, wherein the extreme positions lack foundation—regardless how high or low. The middle way, the path of moderation, is THE way. The middle way is the path of centeredness. When centered, our energy field is vertically aligned; we are aligned with our soul, Heaven and Earth. Aligned with truth. The middle way is sustainable. Extremes are not sustainable. The middle way is the most powerful way, in the long-run.

The middle way makes use of anything that life presents. The middle way is tolerant—and thereby open-hearted. Free of ideas—and thereby open-minded. Without destination—and thereby lovingly detached.

MONEY

Money, like everything else, is an energy. Money flows to and from individuals. Should one cut off the flow of money in either direction, the opposing flow ceases as well. In other words, if a miser cuts spending, then incoming dollars are reduced (*especially if his intention for use of money is* **not** *that of serving others*)

Those who chase after money and security, at the expense of their core truth, shall lose touch with their heart. Obviously money is a means, not an end. It's a tool that can be used to serve others. Or it's a temptation that can be used to serve oneself selfishly. Used for others, it's a godsend. Used for oneself, it's a waste of resources (and a challenging lesson). Money is a flow. The more one directs the flow of money to serving others, the more open the flow of money to oneself.

Right spending serves others. The miser blocks the flow of dollars, both to and from herself. Money is made available to she who follows her heart, given discipline and right action, for the money supports her service.

MORALITY

Morality is an illusion. The moral being believes his/her values are superior to others' values. Thus, morality is based in ego. The moral person believes so strongly in their value system that when others resist, they use *force* to compel others to succumb to their beliefs. Of course, this is ineffective in the long run. Natural law, rather than ego's judgment, determines the societal value of every thing, event, thought, word, and action. The *Tao Te Ching* suggests that the kind man is more effective than the just man. The just man is more effective than the moral man. Why? As kindness (born of compassion) is rooted in the soul, morality is born in the ego, and justice resides between—as it may be rooted in the soul or may be applied by the mind (ego) as a function of societal norms.

MOTHER-INFANT CONNECTION

There is no stronger bond than that between mother and infant. Mother and infant share an energy field. Their aura is one—and must be treated as such. In my experience I have observed that mother and child may see the same visions and experience sensory patterns that reveal similar emotions while experiencing energetic healing. For example, during consecutive energywork/bodywork sessions, both a mother and her five-year old child saw a vertically-bisected purple and green field, with purple to the left as though in front of the left eye and green as though in front of the right eye. To heal a young child, be certain the mother has been healed of the identical issue, or the energy of the child might snap back to the unhealed state, as the mother holds the more influential energetic field (aura). Theory suggests that the *terrible two's* (at two years of age) experienced by babies may occur as the baby is significantly releasing her connection from the etheric world and from the mother's aura, assuming its own aura.

MOVEMENT

The path forward
at times
moves backward.

The Tao prescribes circular movement, including return and yielding, to resolve all that was previously unresolved, to move ahead. Thus the path forward, at times, moves backward.

NATION

When a great nation errs, it realizes its mistake. Corrects the mistake. And admits the mistake. Thus, a great nation acts with sensitivity and integrity. It may be believed by its citizenry and other countries. It recognizes its enemy as nothing more than the shadow it casts itself. Thus, it learns from its enemy how to heal itself. And in so doing, heals its relationship with its enemy. A just country manufactures trucks. An unjust country builds missiles. A balanced country feeds its own people and doesn't meddle in the affairs of other nations. Thereby the country is a beacon to other countries.

The prudent government does not tax too heavily, or it starves its population. It is not too invasive, or its citizens lose their spirit. It always acts on behalf of the people's interests. It trusts its citizens and so it is trusted by its citizens — and so its citizens act with integrity. It does not infringe on the privacy and freedom of the people.

NON-COMPETITION

The greatest athletes or performers compete only with themselves. Thus no one can compete with them. This is non-competition. Perfect competition. The best competitor wants competitors at their best, and competes in the spirit of play, as though a child (e.g., Chicago Bear running back Walter Payton). When competing as a child, rather than from — for example, anger — mental and physical performance are optimized (as blood flow, mental focus and physical resilience are heightened).

(TO) OVERCOME

To overcome
anything,
we must overcome
only ourselves.

The soft overcomes the hard. As an example, consider how water carves even the most stoic rock formations into monumental canyons. The slow overcomes the fast. Recall the renowned race of the tortoise and the hare. Flexibility overcomes rigidity. The yogi maintains perfect posture at a mature age, whereas the aging football player, once of great strength, has a probability of losing physical posture and musculoskeletal function.

To overcome, we must try. We must always try. We must never give up. Never surrender to doubt. One step before the other, we can accomplish anything (within reason) that we focus our intention and effort upon. Each of us is born with inherent challenges that we must overcome. Our so-called imperfections, the challenges we must rise above, are in actuality, perfect. As they cause us to learn fundamental and subtle life lessons.

Paradoxically, to overcome any situation we must initially transcend our inner world (attitude and bodymind energy via *conscious activity*; see *Voice of The Soul: A Call To Action*), after which material world shifts automatically follow. Recall that material manifestation is initiated by inner transformation. To overcome any situation, first we must change our attitude. A positive attitude is the only path to salvation. Of course, this is much easier said than done — as doubt is pervasive. Yet, even in the face of doubt, we must take steps that illustrate our determination and readiness to act on our own behalf (even if we don't believe in ourselves at a specific moment). Take steps as though you do believe, that is, with confidence in the ultimate outcome of the process. And sooner than later, outer circumstances will shift (at least a bit and more so if aligned with your soul's path), affirming that you can do it. You can overcome. Like an effective football running back that is stopped in his tracks after running into a group of tacklers, keep your feet moving, and you might be surprised that you gain further ground. Keep going — and you will advance. Perhaps not quite as quickly as you hope, yet nonetheless, you'll get there.

OWNERSHIP — WITHOUT POSSESSION

See the section on *Love — True Love (Loving Detachment)*.

When ownership regards inanimate objects, employ assets in the highest form of service possible. When you no longer are able to utilize the asset to its highest service (to humanity), sell (or donate) the asset to that individual, group, or organization that can use the asset in the highest way (for humanity).

As an example, I gave a Martin D-15 acoustic guitar, a fine instrument, to a barista who works in a local café, as he is a serious songwriter/guitarist who did not own a guitar, and I had five guitars. The guitar was collecting dust in my studio. First I loaned the guitar to my friend. Then, at Christmas, I gifted him the guitar. He is now playing weekly, and has a great band. His songs have been listed on RollingStone.com. He is using the asset — the guitar — in the highest manner.

PAIN

To alleviate the experience of emotional pain, open your heart. To alleviate physical pain, divert your focus away from the sensation. Emotional pain is an experience that occurs when we are focused upon so-called past or so-called future. Emotional pain does not occur if focused in the present moment — as only ego experiences emotional pain, unlike soul, which is always focused upon the present moment and thus never experiences pain.

The monkeymind experiences pain based upon its anticipatory fear of the future, and based upon prior *mistakes* (actually, there is no such thing as a mistake so long as we learn and master the lessons presented). To the bodily aspect of the bodymind, pain is physical sensation experienced by the sensory aspect of the nervous system. Manage physical pain as recommended by a professional.

A holistic approach to pain management follows:

Feel the pain in its physical totality, inhaling into the region at progressively deeper levels, exhaling the sensation up to the Universe (a la Qi Gong-based therapeutic breathwork). Deal with the core mental beliefs that link pain with dysfunctional (painful) body-held emotions (primarily in the internal organs and, secondarily, in all cells) and psycho-energetic blockages throughout the body.

Focus upon the present moment rather than so-called past or future.

Pain has a limit. It is a finite quantity. Should one continue to breathe and focus progressively deeper into the region experiencing pain, the individual may find that there is an end to the feeling, a point beneath which there is no additional pain. The person shall find that this energy may be *sent up* ("Beam me up, Scotty!") to the Universe. Since we are holistic beings — comprised of body and mind — the mind must also be dealt with. Mental awareness may be addressed by reading or receiving psychological therapy focused upon the emotions and emotional reactivity. In turn, reactivity is anticipatory (expected in the future) and may be based, in part, upon past patterns of reactivity. Focus upon pain begets further pain. Don't focus on pain. Don't empower pain. Breathe and think positive! Now, all of this advice, these aforementioned steps, should not be followed rigidly or dogmatically. It is still advisable to consult a medical professional in order to determine if there is some medical condition that should be taken into account in your own particular situation.

PATIENCE

> *Patience is the ultimate test of faith.*
> *When impatience strikes you,*
> *do you still reach for natural order (a.k.a. God)?*
> *Do you surrender to whatever bounty She may provide?*
> *Or do you obsess upon a desired outcome*
> *and resist natural order?*

> *Rushing ahead,*
> *we do not go far,*
> *we do not succeed,*
> *we miss the natural rhythm,*
> *we block natural order's (God's) will and cadence*
> *and fail to learn the lesson.*

Can you be still as long as it takes to experience the *mud* (in your mind) settling to the bottom of psyché? What does this mean? Our conscious and subconscious aspects contain energetic impurities. When we quiet (i.e., *transcend*) the mind through meditation, we allow impurities to release, rendering clarity.

Life is easy when everything's going your way. But, when the chips are down, can you remain patient—i.e., do you maintain complete faith and thereby neither worry nor try to rush a desired outcome? Or do you notice you become impatient? Impatience and intolerance are classic symptoms of a closed heart chakra (in traditional Chinese medicine). So, patience requires an open heart. Which is fueled by faith. So, patience requires faith. Faith that higher power will provide what we truly need (which may vary from egoic desires). Higher power knows exactly what we need, and will present us with exactly that—so we may learn the precise lesson commensurate with our juncture in life.

The *Tao Te Ching* states that the three great virtues are simplicity, compassion, and patience. Typically, the more significant the lesson, the more challenging the tests for mastery. Patience requires an open heart — empowered by faith. Faith that we will receive exactly what we need, and thus we can trust in higher power (eternally). So, patience is the ultimate test of faith.

Since faith is perhaps the ultimate lesson, and patience is a challenging test of faith, many life processes are designed to be slow (S - L - O – W), so as to require patience; change is slow (S - L - O – W) by design, to present tests of patience and, thereby faith. *If we could manifest everything we desired instantly, we would not be presented with an opportunity to master the lesson of patience.*

Can you remain *unmoving* until the right action arises by itself (via unforced natural order)? Can you sit still, in the face of impatience, all the while trusting higher power to provide precisely what you need — but on higher power's time schedule (which is designed to test our patience!)?

In other words, can you practice non-action (See the section entitled *Action – Non-Action*) in the face of adversity, trusting that if you merely do work to raise your state of consciousness, that you will magnetically attract the precise lesson (including props in the form of specific people, objects and events) that you need at this precise time to evolve?

PATRIOTISM

pa-tri-ot [or, esp. Brit., **pat-ri-ot**], noun.
1. a person who loves, supports, and defends his or her country and its interests with devotion.
2. a person who regards himself or herself as a defender, especially of individual rights, against presumed interference by the federal government.

Patriotism is necessary only when a country experiences chaos (separatism, non-unity) — either from inside or from an international source. Promote intra-national and inter-national harmony to preclude the need for patriotism. It is best to have no need for patriotism. If patriotism is necessary, it should be practiced with an intention of universal unity and resultant peace.

PEACE — INNER PEACE

We experience inner peace when we are free of egoic desire and judgment (i.e., we *accept* rather than resist the natural flow of life).

PEACE — WORLD PEACE

If the world's leaders are centered in the Tao, there is harmony, as laws are written from the heart — in a loving and trusting manner. War is not necessary. Unity and cooperation between countries attempt to halt world hunger, global warming, world disease and other pervasive issues. *Not to be confused with whirled peas.*

PERSEVERING

Prepare as extensively as possible. The late, great Chicago Bears running back Walter Payton was said to workout longer and harder than all other NFL players. So he developed into one of the greatest football players in history. My grandfather's friend, Dr. Benjamin Boshes, Chair of Northwestern University Medical School's Department of Neurology, hailed the *prepared mind*. Proactively research your objective. What does the task require? What resources do you need to most efficiently and effectively perform the task? Do your work beforehand to make the actual performance as graceful and effortless as possible. Persevere, be patient, have faith. Mt. Everest is conquered one step at a time. Maintain focus in each moment. Give each moment your best effort. To persevere is to be completely focused in the present moment — understanding that for every step you take, natural order (the Universe) will take ten steps to support your effort (as long as aligned with natural order, your soul's highest path).

PRAYER

We can influence the effectiveness of prayer. Grounded body-centered-prayer using breath, intention, and sacred language (sacred geometry) may turbo-charge the power of prayer, as we are a complete energetic circuit when literally grounded, centered, and unified (i.e., connected to the wisdom of Heaven and Earth). What does this mean? As described in the section entitled *Antahkarana*, our energetic system is like that of a light bulb. We must have positive and negative (ground) polarities flowing through us to be a complete energetic circuit—a complete bodymind. When we are focused merely in mind, we (and thereby our prayer) are not as complete as when we are focused in body and mind.

This may be accomplished through the simple exercise of abdominal breathing—focusing the mind's attention on physical feeling of the rise and fall of the lowest portion of the abdomen (diaphragmatic expression of the breath in the lower torso). In this way we ground prayer in Heaven and Earth through guided breathing. When we pray, we speak to the Infinite. Offer prayer, then let the thought go.

When we meditate, the Infinite speaks. We can further enhance the power of prayer by using mantra (sonic *sacred geometry*) based in ancient, sacred languages that have stood the test of time (including Tibetan, Chinese, Aramaic, Sanskrit, and Hebrew—languages created using sacred phonetics) or, more so, through direct use of sacred phonetics—which is the language that higher power hears most easily. [See the section entitled *Sacred Geometry*.]

PRESENCE

To be present is to focus the mind's attention on the present moment. This is tantamount to mindfulness. The soul focuses only upon the present moment. Ego focuses only upon so-called past and future. To be present is to be aligned with the soul. Presence is the ultimate condition—as when present we access the wisdom and energy of Heaven and Earth. We are innately guided to highest performance of any task when focused upon the present moment.

PRESUMPTION

Presuming to know is a disease. The ego approaches situations as though it knows what to expect—rather than acknowledging that every moment is unique and new. The wise woman acknowledges that the more she sees, the less she knows. The soul approaches each moment as a new experience and thereby presumes to know nothing. Thus the soul, focused merely in the present moment, does not claim to have prior knowledge (from prior moments—the so-called past) that may be applied to the present moment. To presume is to assume this moment is the same as a prior moment, which it is not. Each moment is new and unique and so presumption is wholly inappropriate.

PROJECTION

See the section entitled *Mirror(ing)*.

PURITY

> *True purity seems impure.*
>
> Tao Te Ching

Why? Recall that to heal we must again feel emotions that earlier we were not ready to process appropriately, and so buried the emotion. To heal we must dig up, reveal and release these emotions. This process allows us to experience an unresolved emotion again, in the hope that this time around it will be properly processed and thereby resolved (healed). This leads to our evolution, our *purification*. Paradoxically, *the process of achieving purity seems impure (again, as we must dig up, re-feel, and release previously buried emotion).*

During energywork practice, I observed that clients initially found it difficult to experience (i.e., feel) pure emotion. They would jumble sadness and anger as though one confusing emotion. In other words, they would inappropriately react to situations that would rationally invoke a reaction of *anger* by expressing sadness, and vice-versa. Given a disciplined healing regimen, the clients eventually experienced pure anger, pure sadness, pure worry, pure fear, pure joy, etc.

100

To heal we must experience pure emotion—for only then may we completely release the emotion from the bodymind and auric field.

PURPOSE

Life purpose is a paradox,
although momentary *purpose may shift,*
an underlying life purpose
pervades each lifetime.

The Master fulfills her purpose in each moment. As she lives in the moment, she lives her purpose each moment, as guided by her soul. She intends, thinks, speaks, and acts from her heart and soul. Her purpose arises in the moment. Her purpose may vary each moment in form, yet in underlying substance is consistent from moment to moment. Her momentary purpose is seeded by unconditional love. *One's life purpose is revealed by the soul, not ego. Life purpose is revealed via intuition, dreams, and synchronicity.* The Master is fed by the wisdom of Heaven and Earth (which supplies infinite information). The master is a channel, a conduit, for such energy in each moment, and thereby fulfills universal will in each moment.

A great paradox encompasses purpose. Although purpose is a moment-to-moment practice, each of us is born with a unique overall purpose that may be *defined as one's core (subconscious) mode of expression* (outward creativity and inward receptivity via the five senses). Each of us is born primarily an artist (visual expression), dancer (kinesthetic expression), or musician (auditory expression). Which of these activities caused you to lose track of time, especially as a kid?

Through the five senses, we receive and express information at the core of our being (i.e., the subconscious mind and core energetic template—described as the Central Channel or Antahkarana). Through information both expressed and received through the five senses, we directly influence the subconscious mind, our inner energetic template, and subsequently our material experience.

In sum, our purpose is to create, via the five senses, to enhance our inner energetic vibration and, thereby, universal energetic vibration (a.k.a. universal consciousness).

RECEPTIVITY (TO TRUTH)

The *Tao Te Ching* states that when a receptive (sensitive) person hears higher truth, she immediately embodies truth. When an average person encounters higher truth, she half believes, half doubts it. When a fool hears higher truth, she laughs aloud. If she didn't laugh, it wouldn't be higher truth!

We receive information, which may affect us superficially (conscious mind predominantly) or may affect us deeply (conscious mind and subconscious mind). Some information may predominantly affect the subconscious mind (via information received through the five senses).

We receive information through varied mechanisms. We receive higher truth through the five senses — which serve as a direct gateway (portal) to the subconscious energetic template. Thus receipt of higher truth is a bodily (bodymind) experience.

RELATIONSHIP

Relationship is a paradox simply described by the mechanics of a Venus Flytrap plant. A Venus Flytrap plant has two primary functional mechanisms. Beautiful nectar, and jaws. The nectar represents the superficial beauty that attracts us to another being (physical, mental, emotional and/or spiritual connection). The jaws represent the lessons that the relationship presents to us. *Paradoxically, the reason for relationship is to learn lessons, not simply to enjoy the enticing nectar.* [For a detailed explanation, see Volume 2 in the *Anatomy of the Human Fabric* Trilogy entitled *Conscious Relationship*.]

Recall that the primary reason underlying our existence, in simplest terms, is *to learn*. We are here to master life's lessons, both fundamental and progressively subtle. To expedite the process, we participate in relationship with other beings. Specific rules govern relationship:

1. **Initial Compatibility**. Pursuant to the Venus Flytrap analogy, the nectar of the other person initially attracts us to engage in relationship, either platonic or romantic, with another person. Initial compatibility predominates the initial (approximate) ninety days of the dynamic between the parties.

2. **Ninety-Day Rule**. At approximately ninety days into a relationship, the dynamic shifts from a mostly conscious (superficial) dynamic to a substantial subconscious dynamic — wherein the shadow aspect of the subconscious mind initially appears at the surface. In other words, at ninety days we see the *other side* of the personality of the person we relate to. Using the Venus Flytrap analogy, the nectar of the other person holds us in relationship to the other person. The nectar must be enticing enough to hold our attention for approximately ninety days and beyond so we don't run away when *the fit hits the shan*. The jaws close ever-so-slowly and take approximately ninety days to shut — at which time the shadow aspect of the subconscious personality, the *other* side of one's personality, reveals itself.

3. **Triggering**. The only way to heal is to re-experience (re-*feel*) emotion that we weren't ready to feel prior. So, we need something (someone) to trigger us to re-feel similar emotions to those we had buried earlier (at a core, subconscious level). Relationship provides this opportunity as, at approximately ninety days, we subconsciously trigger one another to feel. In other words, we trigger one another to *feel* subconsciously and to *react* consciously. More specifically, we trigger the subconscious aspect of one another's personalities to re-experience previously buried emotions, and react.

4. **Shadow Compatibility**. Pursuant to the Venus Flytrap analogy, the interplay of the reactivity of two individuals is a very healing process. And, how well two people communicate and process — as though a team — is a barometer of the strength of the healing force of the relationship, which in this context is termed shadow compatibility. In other words, when two individuals are triggered to react emotionally, *the ability to work through their (reactive) emotions in a synergistic way is a*

measure of their compatibility. Initial compatibility is based solely upon the superficial power of *nectar*. Shadow compatibility is the measure of how well the *couple* can communicate and process together when the *fit hits the shan*. The purpose is not necessarily for the couple to stay together. *The purpose is for each individual to gain self-awareness through the dynamic interaction with the other individual. If appropriate, the couple will stay together. If not, the couple will recognize that they have learned all lessons possible, and move on to the next learning experience.*

5. **Transcendent Compatibility**. Following the stages of Initial Compatibility and Shadow Compatibility, a couple may concurrently pursue a relationship with heightened consciousness (through spiritual/religious connection). Through such engagement they may mutually transcend the personality/ego plane and meet one another on the soul plane. The objective of this path is to receive "direct experience" of the Absolute. To this effect, note that meditation may be a physical experience beyond imagination. Whatever we focus upon in the moment is all we are. Thus, if we focus upon heightened conscious in the moment, we are heightened consciousness. In this manner we become unconditional love—as we focus upon unconditional love when focused upon the infinite source.

In sum, two individuals meet and choose to continue to relate (over time) based upon the power of one another's superficial nectar, the superficial magnet that initially attracts the participants to one another. For example, a boss and employee will meet, via contract, and keep working together as long as the relationship serves not only the company (from a superficial perspective) but also one another—from a deeper perspective. That is, although they work together to receive a paycheck, they also trigger one another's subconscious emotional issues, helping one another to heal.

Note that from the perspective of the monkeymind (lower mind/ego), lessons may be pleasant or not-so-pleasant. Through relationship, parties to a relationship may learn about addiction, betrayal, trust, abundance, lack, joy, teamwork, isolation, harmony, peace, abandonment, engulfment, bliss, etc. In contrast, from the perspective of the soul, all lessons are positive (i.e., "all conditions are favorable!"—The Meditation Master Who Prefers to Remain Nameless) — since all experiences help us to grow (as long as we choose to observe, understand and master the lesson).

RELIGION

Religion is not to be confused with spirituality.
Religion is a human construct.
Spirituality is simply natural belief in a benevolent higher power.

Religious practice is tantamount to ritual centered upon a spiritual framework. Religion is a human construct. Spirituality is a natural sense of a good-natured higher power. Of course, no religion is better than any other — especially as all began with a foundation predicated upon the similar fundamental spiritual truths.

RESIDENCE

In this age of skyscrapers, it is best to live close to the ground. Why? To maintain an energetic connection to Earth. [See the section entitled *Grounding* for further explanation.] Recall that the ancient Taoists believed that we gain vital life force from our connection to the energy of Heaven and Earth. Proximity to the Earth helps us maintain this vital connection. Life in a skyscraper surrounds the tenant with electrical wiring, steel, and concrete, overhead and below that may block healthy grounding energy.

When choosing a residence, listen to your intuition about how the place *feels*. Does it feel warm and inviting? cold and stagnant? It can take up to six months to feel comfortable in a new dwelling. Be certain your gut feeling is positive. If not, find another residence.

It may be helpful to consult a feng shui template to determine the energetic characteristics of a potential home. Feng shui is the study of energetic patterns applied to a residence. The ancient Taoist belief is that a house has eight main sectors. Be certain the home you are considering has effective placement of the eight sectors. Then consider placement of furniture in the home by using principles of feng shui to optimize energy flow throughout the home.

An optimal home holds balanced energy—i.e., with energy of the four elements (Earth, Fire, Water, Air) in harmony. Perhaps this explains why a house located adjacent to a natural source of water is so valuable—particularly if the surrounding land has trees (an extension of Earth) yet access to direct sunlight (and good ventilation). Yet, in the alternative, a house not near water or without trees can be a wonderfully balanced home if one consults principles of feng shui.

RESPECT

Paradoxically,
to earn the respect of others,
we must first respect ourselves.
And to respect others,
we must first respect ourselves.

To respect ourselves, we must *be ourselves*—i.e., think, speak, and act in a manner aligned with the truth of who we really are at the core. We must view ourselves without comparison or competition. If we believe in ourselves, others innately believe in us, too. If we believe in ourselves, we are *believable*. We needn't try to convince others. If we are content, we do not seek the approval of others. If we accept ourselves, the world accepts us. If we accept ourselves, we are able to respect all components of the world—as we naturally project our respectful perspective onto others we relate to.

RITUAL

Ritual is the foundation of true faith. At a core level, we need structure: "psyché requires rhythm for growth" (Jack Miller, Ph.D.). *Repetition inspires transformation.* We may unlock and release subconscious blockages through repetitive thoughts, words and actions. Appropriate ritualistic behavior—sacred repetition (wherein the term "sacred" refers to a phenomenon that directly affects the subconscious mind—connects us to the higher self.

Paradoxically, the *Tao Te Ching* describes ritual as *the beginning of chaos*. Why? Because ritual innately accelerates our transformation. To evolve, we must heal. To heal, we must dig up buried emotions that earlier we were not ready to resolve. To do so, we attract props (people, objects, and events) that will trigger us to feel once more the emotions that we buried long before. This may feel like chaos — yet is actually perfectly aligned with natural order, as it promotes opportunities for eventual enhanced self-awareness (evolution).

SACRED GEOMETRY

Sacred geometry refers to external agents that **directly** *affect the subconscious mind (via the five senses).* The five physical senses are able to discern subtle variations in the quality of stimuli. For example, the visual sense is able to distinguish distinct shapes and colors; the auditory sense is able to discern distinct musical notes; the kinesthetic sense is able to discern distinct movements; the olfactory sense is able to distinguish odors; and the gustatory sense is able to discern distinct tastes.

A stimulus is described as *sacred* **if it is specifically recognized by the subconscious mind and has direct significant impact upon the subconscious energetic template.** Only specific stimuli profoundly and deeply affect the subconscious template. It is as though *primordial shapes, colors, sounds, odors, movements, and tastes are pre-programmed into the awareness of the subconscious mind and serve as keys to unlock the subconscious template — accelerating healing and evolution.* The term *geometry* refers to the subconsciously-identifiable distinct form of a given stimulus.

Sacred geometry takes five forms — each identified by one of the five physical senses. Visual sacred geometry is based upon shape and color. Auditory sacred geometry is based upon tone, rhythm and syllabic content (e.g., mantra). Kinesthetic sacred geometry is based upon variations in movement. Olfactory sacred geometry is based upon variations in odors. Gustatory sacred geometry is based upon variations in tastes.

As an example, five alphabets are considered to be sacred (geometry). The specific shapes of the letters are recognized by the subconscious mind. These letters (shapes) serve to unlock subconscious blockages.

For this reason these alphabets, Aramaic, Tibetan, Chinese, Sanskrit, and Hebrew have stood the test of time.

Another example is mantra. Mantras are an ancient series of syllables that are spoken aloud. The syllables are largely based upon vowel sounds. Specific vowel sounds affect the subconscious mind (and internal organs) in different ways. The vowel sound "AHHH" opens the heart chakra (energetic center); "HOOO" opens the spleen, pancreas, and stomach (releasing worry); "WO" releases fear from the kidneys; beyond vowels, "SHHH" releases anger from the liver and gall bladder; and "SSS" releases sadness and sorrow from the lungs. These syllables also deeply affect the subconscious mind.

As an example of sacred movement, the asanas (postures) of yoga, and positions of t'ai chi, are recognized by, and have profound effect upon, the subconscious mind.

SCARCITY

Scarcity is an illusion of the personality. From the perspective of the soul, we are always given precisely what we *need* in each moment—for the purpose of learning, healing and evolving. We are given what we *want* (from the perspective of the ego) only if this is aligned with our soul's evolution.

The stronger our belief that higher power will guide us to abundance, the greater the probability that we will be given what we want … or better! Conversely, a belief system of lack will manifest as material lack. So, have faith that higher power will give you exactly what is appropriate—and that is precisely what you will receive.

The ability to let go ("Let go, let God"), a demonstration of faith, enhances the odds of receipt of abundance (if aligned with your soul's evolutionary path). Faith is a fundamental lesson we must learn. When we have faith, we are granted material abundance if aligned with our evolution. Lack of faith (or karmic repercussion) results in material scarcity.

(THE) SEEKER

Let go of the need to seek
And truth shall be revealed

Divine truth is eternally available to the soul, but not to ego. Soul focuses solely upon the present moment. It does not exist in so-called past or future. Conversely, ego focuses only upon so-called past and future. It cannot exist in the present moment. So, truth is available only to the soul, as highest truth can be accessed only when focused in the present moment. If we consciously seek — focusing on so-called future — from the perspective of the ego (monkeymind), we block the possibility of access to truth. We must let go of focus on the so-called future to access truth, via the soul, which is available to us every moment, if we so choose (via conscious activity which inspires enhancement of the inner voice — not via thinking). The ego seeks — focusing on the so-called future. The soul, focused upon the present moment, not seeking future gain, innately accesses truth (eternally).

The seeker ever shall seek. The meditator ever shall find.

SELF-AWARENESS

We are not the ego (monkeymind). We are soul. If we define ourselves through external associations, we cannot know who we truly are. We shift in each moment, thus any identification with externalities is both false and limiting. Self-awareness infers understanding of the core self and superficial personality. To gain self-awareness, we must learn through experience. To be self-aware is to identify our unique life purpose and life service innately, and to understand that our true self is unified with soul (and the present moment), not ego (and focus upon so-called past/future).

SENSES — THE PHYSICAL SENSES

The *Tao Te Ching* recognizes that the physical senses may be considered from two perspectives. There are superficial aspects of the physical senses — connected to ego. And there are sublime aspects to the physical senses—connected to soul. As such, the *Tao Te Ching* paradoxically states that colors blind the eyes, sounds deafen the ears, and flavors numb the taste-buds. This infers that the material aspects of the five senses are superficial—and so are virtually meaningless and purposeless (to the point of being deleterious to our evolution—as they may distract us from attaining self-awareness). Thus, focus upon the external senses is a futile practice. The *Tao Te Ching* recommends focus upon deeper insight available through meditation, via the inner eye (and inner senses).

And yet, paradoxically, the physical senses are critical to the process of evolution, as they are a direct portal to the subconscious template. They are keys that unlock subconscious blockages. We express and receive through the five physical senses. A powerful practice to shift subconscious blockage is to *engage one or more of the physical senses while focused upon real-time emotion.* For example, if you are frustrated with something (i.e., feeling anger), go for a run while feeling the emotion. Kick the pavement, run faster and harder when you feel more anger. Breathe. Exhale the anger. The anger will release from your bodymind and auric field at an accelerated pace. Dance whatever emotion you feel for twenty minutes per day for a healthy release of emotion. Listen to music that supports the emotion you dance—so you receive through the auditory sense and express through the kinesthetic sense. In this way you can accelerate the unlocking of blockages from the subconscious template. Similarly, expression through any of other senses while feeling real-time emotion is cathartic. [See the section entitled *Creativity.*]

SEPARATION

Separation is an illusion. The soul recognizes that separation is not real, since the soul is aware that all is one. Everything, at a fundamental (energetic) level is unified. For example, if an electron were to pass through the room in which you sit, it would see everything as the same—as everything simply consists of homogenous electrons, protons and neutrons. In fact, odds are staggeringly high that the electron would fly through the room without colliding with anything—as molecules are mostly space. Only ego believes in separation. Ego is not aware of connection to anything else. Ego feels separation as though a very real phenomena.

Yet, this is illusion. We are connected to one another and higher power. In all moments. Since the soul is aware of this truth, we simply need to tap into soul to feel unity (and dissolve the false perception of separation). In other words, presence dissolves an illusory sense of separation. Each of us came from a common source. Each of us shall return to the common source. In theory we are never separated from natural order and infinite unconditional love, so long as we are focused in the present moment (i.e., aligned with the soul).

SERVICE

We are born to serve. Others. The Earth. The Universe. Each of us is born with a unique life service and life purpose. How can we determine our life service? In one of three ways. Either one simply has an innate feeling regarding how to serve; one can determine their appropriate service through trial-and-error activity; or one can enhance the inner voice to reveal appropriate service via a regimen of disciplined conscious activity [see the section Action—Non-Action and *Voice of the Soul: A Call to Action*]. Arguably, although each moment is new—and thus appropriate service could arguably shift from moment to moment, *each of us is born with an over-riding life service*. Our challenge is to determine our highest life purpose and life service. To do so most of us must find a way to enhance the inner voice such that it shall reveal our right path (purpose and service). Note that *the thinking mind cannot ascertain our right purpose and service.*

Our *life purpose benefits us. Life purpose* regards the practice of our core creativity: this is core expression through one (or more) of the five physical senses. This discipline *benefits us*—as it feels good to create from a core level (it enhances our energetic vibrational frequency and, thus, is cathartic). In contrast, our *life service benefits others* and the world. As an example, I have a friend whose purpose is playing violin, yet his service is helping people care for their dogs (he owns a doggy daycare facility).

We may gain clarity regarding our unique life service (and life purpose) by practicing non-action (conscious activity)—which enhances the whisper of the inner voice of truth through dreams, intuition and synchronicity. [See *Action – Non-Action.*] The whisper of the soul, heard via dreams, intuition and/or synchronicity—no accessibly via the thinking mind—will innately guide you to your primary life service.

(TO) SHRINK

To reduce something, or let go of something, we must first allow it to flourish. Only then will we learn the lessons presented by the situation—the reason for our participation in the situation—after which we can release the relationship. If we do not allow the situation to fully expand, we will not learn the lesson(s), and will be required to repeat a similar situation later, to learn these lesson(s).

SIMPLICITY

> *Simplicity, patience and compassion are the three great Virtues.*
>
> *Tao Te Ching*

Truth is always simple. If something isn't simple, it isn't at the level of truth. Resolve situations that don't feel truthful (i.e., simple). If the situations remain untruthful (i.e., not simple), eventually release the situations. More appropriate situations will be presented that will further learning—and will seem simpler (and eventually will feel more comfortable).

To live most simply, recognize that what we *desire* isn't necessarily the same as what we *need*. The ego's desires are limitless. The ego's desires will never be satisfied. In contrast, the soul's needs are always satisfied as the Tao provides the props (people, objects and events) necessary to further our learning (evolution). Hold unwavering faith that this is true—in every moment the Tao will always provide precisely what you need for most efficient and complete evolution.

Observe animals. Animals live simple lives. They eat, they reproduce, and they love. When unfettered in a natural habitat they seem … happy! When the lives of animals are made more complicated, when humans tamper with their natural ways, they become unhappy. For example, I share time with a Rottweiler (a rescue dog) who is now a very loving dog. Yet Rotts are notorious for being savage animals. This is not their natural way. This is a manner imposed by humans who want guard-dogs and promote aggressiveness in the animals. My friend the Rott was raised to be a guard-dog, and then was abandoned to the largest dog pound in Chicago — where Rotts, Dobermans and Pitbulls are not atypically terminated; purportedly 10,000 dogs per year are killed. I found her at the pound and gave her a loving home. After a short time she became trusting and outwardly loving. She is no longer asked to carry out a relatively complex task — being a guard-dog — that is contrary to her true nature. She regained a simple way of being. A simple life. Which is aligned with her true nature. Which seems to agree with her as judged by her perpetual smile. Additionally, a month ago I listened to a report on National Public Radio that somehow documented that Mexican dogs are *happier* than American dogs (and so unhappy American dogs were co-mingled with Mexican dogs to learn how to be happy). The study inferred that the Mexican dogs lived in simpler environments — could this be why they (and presumably their human companions) found relative happiness?

SLEEP

Sleep is as essential as food. Just as specific parameters are required for a healthy diet, sleep should be an equally regimented routine. Prehistoric humans, like animals, slept when it was dark, and hunted, gathered, ate, and communed during daylight hours. Such a schedule is aligned with the timing (biorhythm) of our energetic channels (12 internal organ energy meridians described in Traditional Chinese Medicine). Each internal organ is activated twice per day — every twelve hours — at precisely the same time each day.

The body creates yang (fire element) energy beginning at midnight — to prepare the body for activity later in the morning, so that our inner fire is burning brightly by the time we are programmed to wake — at sunrise. Yang fire builds until 12 p.m. (noon) after which the internal furnace virtually shuts down, allowing yang energy to decrease (yin to increase) so we can sleep after the sun sets.

Sleeplessness not atypically occurs due either to a restless spirit (disturbed "shen") or too much yang energy in one's system (due to caffeine, anxiety, etc.). Anger (fire element) blocks sleep, so be certain to release anger (in healthy ways such as working out, dancing, and/ or painting and creating music about the anger, or other emotional issues — while experiencing real-time emotion). [See *Emotional Release*.] Sleep allows the bodymind an opportunity to re-charge itself and allows psyche to dream — to work out subconscious issues.

Note that the more proficient and frequent one's meditation, the less sleep one needs (as meditation also revitalizes the bodymind). As an example, when I was meditating with a great Hindu master (The Meditation Master Who Prefers to Remain Nameless), I needed no more than three hours of sleep per night.

SOUL

Regardless how caustic one's personality,
beneath is a diamond,
shimmering, radiant, perfect:
the soul.

The soul is perfect. Omniscient. Connected to Heaven and Earth, the Infinite. Eternal. Eternally connected to the Infinite. And yet, in so many moments of most lives (if not all moments); the soul remains hidden — behind the veil of ego. To evolve, we must pierce ego's veil. How do we escape the gravitational pull of ego? By implementing conscious activity combined with positive, self-aware thought. [See *Voice of the Soul: A Call to Action.*]

Soul is aligned with truth. Soul focuses only upon the present moment. In contrast, ego can focus only upon so-called past or future. Soul is tantamount to presence (mindfulness focused only upon presence). Highest truth is accessed only through the present moment. So, soul accesses highest truth. Ego resides in so-called past and future—both of which do not provide reliable information (so-called past is merely one's subjective perception of prior events and so-called future is speculative).

In theory, soul is aligned with what Taoists describe as Heaven and Earth—universal and grounding energies, respectively. We tap Heaven and Earth energies when present (mindful of the present moment). We become a conduit of Heaven and Earth when connected to soul—when focused upon the present moment.

Soul is the true self. In theory, soul travels from lifetime to lifetime, gaining mastery of fundamental and progressively subtle life lessons—until such time as the soul masters life's lessons—and so no longer needs to tread upon the karmic wheel (i.e., no longer returns to the cycle of lifetimes—as the soul has mastered all lessons available on the earth plane).

SOUL THREADS

Everything is connected. All energies are inter-connected. So, we are connected to everything. And, especially, to other people—especially those we deal with on a somewhat regular basis.

We connect to others via energetic threads—invisible channels (cords) of energy that connect via heart and third-eye (pineal gland) connections (a.k.a. Spheres of Influence of the Antahkarana - see the section entitled *Antahkarana*).

These soul threads connect us to everything. Heart threads connect us to sources of vital life force. Third-eye threads connect us to higher intelligence and consciousness. When we sleep, the heart threads remain intact and pineal gland connections sever. When we drop the body (when we die; i.e., soul lets go of the body), we sever both heart threads and pineal gland threads.

Soul threads are also referred to as Spheres of Influence. [See *Antahkarana*.]

SPIRITUALITY

A spiritual being is loving.
Period.
Nothing more, nothing less.
In each moment.

Spirituality is not to be confused with religious practice. Yet, para-doxically, spiritual belief is the original source of the great religions.

Spirituality is, simply, belief in, and reverence for, the absolute source of all things (a.k.a. natural order, the Absolute, higher power, Light, Love, etc.). Thus, the essence of virtually all religions is the same — as they are based upon a common source. Spiritual practice is reverence for absolute essence. Religious practice is adherence to human-con-structed rules and ideas — rather than natural essence and natural law.

A spiritual being is loving. Period. Spirituality is a moment-to-moment practice. In one moment we may focus upon soul. In another moment, by default, we may focus upon ego. Truly spiritual beings access (are sourced by and aligned with) their soul. The soul is con-nected to the infinite source. The soul is always loving. So, if an individual isn't intending, speaking, or acting in a loving manner at any moment, their spiritual practice (focus) is negligible at that time.

STOP

Knowing when to stop,
one can avoid any danger.

Tao Te Ching

"Even a grouper wouldn't get caught
if it kept its mouth shut."
Keevan Sadock (My Grandfather)

Knowing when to stop is as important as knowing when to engage. In every moment we make choices. We choose whether to initiate, continue, or stop any thought, word, and action in each moment.

When should we stop? When the detriment of continuing a thought, word, or action exceeds the benefit (not simply with regard to self but with regard to the world and universe). Recall that love is supporting another on their highest path in all moments. When intention, words, and/or actions do not support the highest path of another in any moment, then stop. One should engage activity fully. And *one should stop fully* — once the decision has been made to stop. In subsequent moments, one may then choose to re-engage, begin anew or do nothing.

Note that *less is more* when initiating activity — especially during the initial ninety-day period (as trust takes ninety days to establish at a fundamental level). In any moment we may stop activity — but with regard to relationship, unless glaring "deal-breaker" factors are obvious (tantamount to abuse — be it physical or emotional), there may be benefit by sticking around — to learn whatever lesson the interpersonal dynamic may present. When in relationship, *do not stop (dis-engage) before the lesson is learned* (unless the dynamic is abusive). Once all lessons of a dynamic are mastered, it is appropriate to stop momentarily, reassess, re-engage, start anew, or do nothing.

Finally, if your intuition tells you to stop, then stop. Always heed the whispers of the inner voice.

STEADFASTNESS

> *To be steadfast is to be aligned*
> *with one's highest self*
> *in each moment.*
> *Steadfastness is a paradox*
> *as steadfastness is constant*
> *and yet steadfastness is change.*
> *It is constant change.*
> *Steadfastness appears change-able*
> *as change is the nature of the Universe.*

Steadfastness is an oxymoron. It is constant change — as change is the nature of the Universe. To be steadfast is to be adaptable to the change that occurs in each moment. Each moment is new. Each moment is unique—differentiated from the moment before. From a core perspective, steadfastness is constant—to be steadfast is to be aligned with one's highest self in each moment. Yet from a superficial perspective, steadfastness appears change-able. To maintain highest alignment, one must adapt to one's changing environment in each moment.

STRENGTH—PHYSICAL STRENGTH

Physical strength is not a function of muscle. Rather, it is a function of connective tissue and *shen* (internal energy) in conjunction with muscular capacity. So, strength is a function of energy.

STUDY—CONSCIOUS STUDY

Conscious study is disciplined, systematic, and focuses upon soul-aligned content. In the words of my grandfather's fishing partner, the late Dr. Benjamin Boshes, Professor Emeritus at Northwestern University Medical School, the "prepared mind" requires disciplined proactive preparation. The prepared mind requires mental workouts that progressively build the strength of intellectual capacity and ability. Any person can build the strength of their mental faculties. Equal in importance to disciplined, preparatory mental workouts is the choice of what subject matter we focus upon. *Focus upon content aligned with the evolution of the soul.* If we choose to focus upon information that is not aligned with the evolution of the soul, we are not engaged in the practice of conscious study.

The prepared mind (a.k.a. bodymind) is a sponge for highest vibration energy. In turn, the bodymind expresses itself (conveys highest vibration) through highest service to benefit the world. Highest study acquires knowledge—in the brain—and transcribes knowledge into wisdom in the body [see the section entitled *Intelligence*]. Such conscious wisdom is transcribed into worldly service.

At times we are *forced* to read information that is not of conscious content. If so, try to bring "light" to the text by remaining aware of how this information might benefit others — i.e., focus upon how this information might be of service to the world.

In sum, conscious study begets conscious knowledge. Conscious knowledge begets conscious wisdom (when integrated into the bodily aspect of the bodymind – as wisdom is mental knowledge that is integrated into the body via *hands-on* experience). Conscious wisdom renders conscious service.

SUCCESS

> *Success is as challenging as failure*
> *as whether up a ladder*
> *or down,*
> *the position is unstable.*
>
> Tao Te Ching

The danger of success is: ego. True, pure success — which serves to benefit the world in the highest way — feeds the soul. False success — which benefits merely the self — feeds the ego, bolstering false pride and blind ambition. *Pure success benefits others*, not simply the individual. True success is the outcome of soul-aligned service. False success is the result of selfish efforts intended simply to benefit oneself.

And yet, even service that benefits others can tempt ego. Thus, it is essential to intend benefit to others — yet do so in a quiet manner, so as to succeed without taking credit and, to succumb from seeing oneself as above others.

The beauty of true success is that it is contagious. So, lead by example. Succeed in a pure, quiet manner and serve as an example to others to do the same.

TAKING

To receive fully, first allow the *thing* (be it a person, object, or event) to be fully given to you. Do not take something before it is offered to you — or receipt of the item shall be incomplete in the long-run.

TALK

> *Those who talk,*
> *don't know.*
> *Those who know,*
> *don't talk.*

Tao Te Ching

Ever notice that some people seem to speak just for the sake of speaking—although they have little to say? This may occur as some people obtain (false) energy from human attention (vampirism). Yet, the individual whose personality is aligned with (focused upon) the soul, receives energy from alignment with Heaven and Earth and, as such, does not seek energy from human interaction (i.e., *attention*).

The individual who is aligned with the soul is aligned with truth—and so does not need to speak simply to receive energy from inter-personal exchange—as she receives more pure and abundant energy from an infinite source.

The purpose of communication is to convey beneficial ideas to others. Nothing more. Nothing less. On a less-is-more basis.

So, speak if you have ideas that somehow may benefit others. Otherwise, quietly align with soul (by employing conscious activity: see Action—Non-Action*), and when thoughts worthy of communication are received, speak.*

When speaking share complete truth, then be silent. Additionally, take a deep (abdominal) breath before speaking—to ground and center thoughts, and to access higher truth (aligned with the soul, Heaven and Earth).

And, from a superficial perspective, consider this question: which speaker seems more believable, a speaker who speaks immediately after being asked a question, or a speaker who waits a moment (i.e., takes a breath), and then answers? The latter speaker seems to have listened to the question, thought about the question deeply, and presents a grounded, strong expression of her opinion.

THINKING (VERSUS FEELING)

The thinking mind cannot access highest truth – such as one's life purpose or life service. Feeling conveys truth. Truth is carried to us by the inner voice that speaks to us internally via dreams and intuition, and externally via synchronicity. *The thinking mind has only questions, the body holds conscious answers.*

THOUGHTS

The *Tao Te Ching* proclaims that one of the three great virtues is simplicity (along with patience and compassion). The simpler your thoughts, the better. Keep to the simple. Truth is always simple. Truth is binary: something is true or not. Keep thoughts to the simple — regardless how complex the situation. Conversely, if thoughts are convoluted and complex, you have not yet recognized truth.

> *Thoughts weaken the mind.*
>
> Tao Te Ching

Paradoxically, the mind is designed to process thought, yet *thoughts weaken the mind*. What does this mean? The *Tao Te Ching* is saying that lower vibration thought, aligned with ego, weakens the mind — which means that *unconscious thoughts distract our attention away from the soul* (and toward ego).

Soul-aligned thought, especially that received through meditation (and conscious activity), bolsters our entire being. So, meditate and *feel* rather than think (in the sense of the egoic aspect of the personality). In any moment we are what we focus upon. Focus upon egoic concepts weakens our being. Focus upon soul-aligned concepts strengthens our being.

Thoughts are powerful — as they create reality. Choose your thoughts carefully. Use affirmation and mantra to retrain the mind to focus upon positivity in each moment. Intention is the basis of spoken word and activity. Intention creates your world. Learn to develop soul-aligned thoughts — so as to create a world beyond imagination.

TIME

Linear time is a human construct designed for our convenience. The clock on the wall expresses linear time so that we can go about our business according to a schedule. Yet, linear time is not real — as all that exists is this moment. And this moment. And this moment. Ad infinitum. So, all that exists is the moment — not a *time* cadence.

From the perspective of the ego, time is finite and, thus, a scarce resource. Yet, from the perspective of the soul, time is infinite as the soul travels from lifetime to lifetime (until mastery of life lessons is achieved — i.e., until there is self-awareness a.k.a. enlightenment).

TIMING

Strike while the iron is hot.
Yet be careful not to burn yourself
by moving too quickly.

Address situations while they are still easy to deal with. Make decisions as soon as your heart is clear. The longer you wait, the more precarious the situation. Details compile and accumulate with time. Decide and act while situations are simple, rather than procrastinate and then deal with a progressively complicated situation. *Yet, do not act until you are absolutely clear regarding the appropriate action to take. To clear yourself, practice soul-aligned activity (non-action and conscious activity).* [See *Action — Non-Action* and *Voice of the Soul: A Call to Action.*]

The body has innate timing mechanisms. The twelve energetic meridians (recognized in acupuncture and Traditional Chinese Medicine) are activated twice per day, once every twelve hours. Our internal organs are activated every twelve hours, in a definite sequence. So, the body is aware of timing (not linear time). Such timing may be described as *biorhythms*. For example, our internal furnace initiates creation of yang (fire, masculine) energy at midnight. Yang energy is created until noon, when yang energy begins to diminish, until midnight, when yang energy is again created. Such a sequence helps us to awaken in the morning (increasing yang energy) and sleep at night (diminished yang energy).

Trust, at a subconscious level, takes approximately ninety days for trust to develop. Until trust is established, less is more. Say and do less, rather than more, until trust is established at a subconscious level. Test this theory — you will be amazed!

Everything transpires in its natural time. Do not force timing. Be patient. Allow situations to arise of their own accord and timing. What is appropriate will present itself at the appropriate time. If we could manifest everything at will, we would not learn the fundamental lesson of patience, so be glad that things take time to develop.

TRANSFERENCE

See the section entitled *Mirror(ing)*.

TRANSFORMATION

> *The path forward*
> *at times*
> *seems to go backward.*

At times, the path forward seems to travel backwards. Why? So we can unbury *prior* unresolved emotion (and energy) stuck in the subconscious energetic template. Sometimes we face experiences that trigger emotion that we're not ready to process (resolve). We then bury these emotions, put off feeling and resolving the emotions to a later time. We sweep the emotion (energy) under the rug (i.e., we bury the emotion in the subconscious mind). To transform and evolve, we must revisit these buried emotions by again feeling similar emotions. To do so, we attract experiences (people, objects, and events) that trigger feelings similar to those we buried in the past.

Transformation takes place in the subconscious and conscious mind. The subconscious mind is said to create (attract) three-quarters of our experience in the world. Again, *we attract experiences that will trigger us to feel emotions similar to those we buried prior. When we resolve these emotions, through healthy avenues of healing, we evolve.*

Transformation (concurrently) takes place in the mind and body. The mind holds thought. The body holds emotion (in the internal organs). Emotion is the body's response to thought. To have transformation, it is not enough simply to resolve conscious thought. We must also shift emotion held in the body. The subconscious mind is efficiently accessed through the body (through movement and other forms of creative expression through the five senses, which are a direct portal to the subconscious energetic template. [See the section entitled *Action – Non-action,* and Volume 3 of *Anatomy of the Human Fabric Trilogy* entitled *Voice of the Soul: A Call to Action.*]

> *One step forward.*
> *Two steps back.*
>
> Anonymous

In theory, transformation can be a graceful process. Yet, in practical terms, the process of transformation – may feel anything but graceful, as we are triggered to feel unresolved emotions again that we were not ready to process appropriately in the past.

To create lasting and transcendent transformation, one must affect not merely the conscious mind but, arguably more significantly, the surrounding and permeating energy matrix (defined as those aspects of the whole of one's being other than conscious mind – including the subconscious mind, aura, and remaining bodymind). Through utilization of ancient philosophy and technology in a systematic and disciplined manner, the guided, individually-tailored process of transformation of self becomes a path of gracefulness and relative effortlessness, rather than a path of toil, suffering, extended duration, and perceived futility resulting in questionable gain.

[See the section entitled *Antahkarana* for a more detailed explanation of transformation (evolution).]

Transformation follows natural rules of evolution. These are alluded to throughout this book, and explained in greater detail in *Voice of the*

Soul: A Call to Action and *Conscious Relationship*. These natural rules include the *Ninety-Day Rule,* phases of energetic development (chakra development every seven years), natural propensity (born artist, dancer, and/or musician) and Antahkarana template—which simply illustrates the *big picture* of transformation. [See the section entitled *Antahkarana.*]

TRUTH

How do you know if something is true? Look inside yourself. Calm your mind through soul-aligned activity (including meditation), then passively hear the whisper of intuition (gut feeling). The whisper of the inner voice speaks through dreams, intuition and synchronicity. We can enhance the voice of inner wisdom through disciplined practice of conscious activity. [See the section entitled *Action: Non-Action.*]

Truth is *always* simple. If something is not simple, in essence, it is not true.

TRUST

How do we help develop a sense of trust (from another person)? Through appropriate focus and reliable, consistent, and supportive conduct over a period of time.

Focus. In any given moment, should we choose to focus upon the precepts of the Tao or enlightened information, we are innately trustworthy (as we are illumined, transparent, and radiant) as our thoughts are (and intention is) trustworthy. With nothing to prove, intention is pure and others innately trust you.

Conduct. Conduct that is familiar and easily and obviously recognizable as familiar, constant, stable, non-threatening, and non-forceful is trustworthy conduct. Act accordingly.

Time. It typically takes approximately ninety days to establish trust at a subconscious level. Until trust is established at a subconscious level, *less is more* — i.e., say and do less rather than more for the initial ninety days of any relationship. Try it ... you will be pleasantly surprised.

Note that if we do not trust others, they become untrustworthy. If we trust others, they innately trust us. Trustworthiness begets trustworthiness.

As an example, the book entitled *The Little Prince* concerns a prince and a fox. The prince hopes to befriend the fox. The fox tells the prince that he is a wild animal and that to tame him he must establish trust. To establish trust the fox asks the prince to sit upon a rock at the horizon and sit there for an entire day, where the fox can see the prince in the periphery. Then each day the prince is to sit a few feet closer to the fox. Over time the fox innately gains trust for the prince — as the prince acts in a constant, stable, non-threatening, nonforceful, and timely manner.

UNCERTAINTY

> *The monkeymind abhors uncertainty.*
> *To thwart uncertainty*
> *the monkeymind takes any action necessary*
> *to gain an illusory sense of control.*

The nature of the universe is entropy. Uncertainty is a constant — and necessary — condition. Why necessary? For without uncertainty — i.e., if everything were certain — we would not learn how to master fundamental life lessons including faith and patience. Uncertainty inspires us to master lessons of faith and patience. [See sections entitled *Faith* and *Patience*.]

To deal gracefully with uncertainty, neither seek nor expect — focus, rather, upon the present moment (not so-called future or so-called past). If we welcome all experiences — as opportunities to learn — we are not rattled by uncertainty. Attempts to control the future are (obviously) futile. "Let go, let God." Trust that right events are unfolding. *Be present.*

Note that there are only two certainties. Natural order (the Absolute, infinite, eternal, etc.) is certain; uncertainty (a.k.a. change) is certain.

UNDERSTANDING

The more you know
the less you understand.

The Master recognizes that entropy (randomness) is the nature of the universe. Each moment creates more questions than answers. The fool, who knows little, thinks he understands a lot (but does not). The Master, who understands much, recognizes that she knows little relative to how much there is to know.

Empathy and compassion are essential if one is to understand other people. Empathy is the ability to feel what another person feels (i.e., to stand in their shoes). Compassion is the understanding that each person holds a perfect, beautiful soul and yet may act from ego at times, the human aspect that over time will evolve. The more one can quiet the static of the mind, the greater their ability to understand innately. The wider one's range of experience, the greater their capacity to understand.

Understanding is wisdom—mental knowledge integrated into the bodily aspect of bodymind. Thus, understanding, like wisdom, is holistic in nature. [See the section entitled *Wisdom*.]

VALUES—SOCIETAL VALUES

Must you value what others value
and avoid what others avoid?
How ridiculous!

Obviously, people are unique. So why do so many people subscribe to homogenous societal values? Is it lack of creativity? Fear of not *fitting in*? Or actual preference? Most likely it's a combination of these factors and not due to the latter factor alone. Peer pressure and a sense of *fitting in* are compelling reasons for many people to surrender to uniformity. Yet, of course, we succumb to peer pressure due to insecurity. Insecurity (ego's fear) drives people to uniformity and homogeneity.

Rather than fall prey to societal values, value what feels right for you. Have the courage to be unique in the face of uniformity. Others will follow suit—i.e., will be their authentic selves—if you lead the way. Respect your unique preferences. Follow them. Honor them. Create a unique path aligned with your truth. And others will respect you. Ignore your truth, disrespect your truth, and others will disrespect you.

VIBRATION

Contemporary quantum physicists have empirically proven that matter and etheric compounds, such as air, are comprised of quantum particles including molecules, atoms, protons, neutrons, and electrons. Scientists have discovered that electrons, essentially particles of light traveling at 186,000 miles per second, vibrate randomly. This vibration within the atom is named "**Brownian motion.**" Western science proved that matter and energy, per se, vibrate. And quantum physicists have objectively proven that we can **consciously alter** vibration.

In a laboratory experiment, water was examined under an electron microscope before and after it was subjected to an emotion that was expressed by a nearby individual. As a result, the water's appearance, strongly suggested that it have been influenced by the emotion of the individual, and was clearly altered. When placed near the expression of love, water takes the shape of an organized crystalline form. When subjected to anger and hatred, the water's crystalline matrix appears disorganized and dull beneath the microscope.

Ancient indigenous cultures, similar to modern quantum physicists, postulated that everything vibrates. They believed that human beings are comprised of vibrating particles. Unlike the empirically substantiated subatomic particles described by contemporary scientists, the ancients believed that we are made of light. Since they believed that light vibrates, they thereby believed that people, comprised of light particles densely linked in the form of matter, vibrate. Further, they theorized that varying degrees of vibration could be found within specific aspects of each individual. And, similar to quantum scientists, they believed that vibration could be *consciously altered*. The ancients believed that higher vibration (relative to a given aspect of the bodymind) was tantamount to health, whereas lower vibration is stagnancy, thereafter disease and, ultimately, death.

VIOLENCE AND WAR

All decent men detest violence and, thereby, weapons of violence and fear. They avoid use of force except in most dire necessity — and then exercise force only with highest restraint.

Enemies are not monsters, but, rather, are humans. So the conscious *combatant* does not wish personal harm, nor does he rejoice in victory. *"How could one rejoice in victory in the slaughter of men? The warrior enters battle gravely, with sorrow and great compassion, as if attending the funeral of a friend."* (Stephen Mitchell, *Tao Te Ching*.) The greatest warrior, the pacifist, understands that one cannot govern by using force, nor can enemies be ultimately defeated through force — as violence always rebounds upon oneself. *Violence: unreasonable and unrational behavior ... the virtual definition of insanity. War is mass insanity.*

WEALTH

Wealth is a state of mind. He is wealthy who believes he has *enough* (to serve others adequately). We accumulate more by giving more — wealth is flow. Thus, the more the master gives, the greater her wealth.

WILL

The master (a term used liberally throughout the *Tao Te Ching* and other ancient texts) surrenders her will to Divine will, thus the master has no will. The master's task is simply to serve in the highest way in each moment. How may we surrender our will? Simply say so ("I surrender my will to God's will.") And so it is! Why is this advantageous? Because we can help others beyond imagination, and thereby serve ourselves, beyond imagination.

We are granted freewill while on the Earth plane — so be careful what you ask for (as you must might receive it!). The question is … where does your preference originate? From ego or soul? To be certain you prefer what is best for the evolution of your soul, *surrender your free will to highest will.*

WISDOM

Wisdom is knowing oneself. It is *bodily-integrated* self-awareness. Paradoxically, true wisdom may seem foolish — from the perspective of the ego. In fact, from the perspective of the ego, truest wisdom may seem childish.

From a technical energetic perspective, wisdom is mental knowledge that integrates into the body *through experience.* We are holistic beings, best understanding each person here as body and mind as a single, integrated unit). We attain knowledge (in the mind), which is transcribed into wisdom (in the body). As an example, consider how we learn a job. Not atypically, it is not enough simply to hear or read instructions — we need to actually act (physically move the body) to *learn* fully and to master the task at hand. Thus, wisdom is mental knowledge that integrates into bodily understanding. We innately glean wisdom by accessing the present moment, which aligns us, via the soul, to the wisdom of Heaven and Earth.

WORDS

Truth is always simple. Thus, true words tend to be less than eloquent. Eloquent words tend not to convey truth efficiently. Words create reality. As do intention and action. Careful what you say. Positive words manifest as positive material outcomes.

Examples of positive words are affirmations and mantra. [See the section entitled *Sacred Geometry.*]

WORK — WORKING HARD VERSUS WORKING SMART

Working hard is merely that. Working hard does not guarantee better results. In contrast, working smart infers more efficient and effective results.

A combination of clear intention and systemic effort support optimal outcome. Excessive effort based upon unclear intention will render somewhat cloudy results; such effort will prove to be either inefficient, ineffective, or both inefficient and ineffective. In contrast, the best intention unsupported by disciplined effort will result in compromised results. Hard work infers great effort, toil, and perceived personal sacrifice. Working smart entails an intention to help not merely oneself but others, a clear vision regarding how to implement a plan, self-understanding of one's strengths and weaknesses, and subsequent effort that is systematic and disciplined.

The epitome of working smart is non-action (to gain clarity) followed by direct action (to gain material outcome). [See the section entitled *Action – Non-Action.*]

Finally, working smart entails one's choice to work at what one enjoys. Do what you love — success will follow. When working, give your full concentration. When not working, let it (your work) go. Just do your job, then let go — for she who remains attached to her work creates nothing that endures.

Why is this true? All that exists is the moment. Things change in each moment. By remaining attached to the work of a prior moment, we miss the essence of work to be created in the present moment (which may be different). And, by remaining attached to work in all moments, we do not relax, meditate, and rejuvenate — we miss the opportunity for revitalization and serenity. We block the voice of Heaven and Earth from working through us, as conduits, to manifest highest creation in subsequent moments. Pour yourself completely into your work. Give it your all. Then, when the work is done, make no claim. Just show the results. Let the results speak for themselves. Let the process of creation remain a mystery (to others).

YIELDING

The way of the Tao is passive. Allow flow. Move when guided by flow. Yield to the moment.

YOUTHFULNESS

The way of vitality
and youthfulness
is flexibility.
Surrender to flow.

The way of death
is rigidity,
resistance to flow.

To remain youthful, practice non-action (gain clarity and self-awareness). Align with flow. Let all come and go effortlessly, without desire. Be graceful in each moment. To do so, do not expect results (or resistant to *what is*) and thus never be disappointed.

The flexible spirit never grows old. View each moment as new, as though experienced for the first time, as from the perspective of an infant.

Further, move the body. Practice core creativity. [See the sections entitled *Creativity* and *Action – Non-Action*. See also the companion book, *Voice of the Soul: A Call to Action*.]

ZERO-SUM GAME

Human energy is finite. Divine energy is infinite. The Tao, the source of all, is infinite. Focus upon the Tao renders infinite energy. Focus upon people renders finite energy. When focused upon people, engaged in interpersonal relationship, you may gain or lose energy — as *the totality of human interaction is a zero-sum game – unless you are concurrently focused upon the Tao*.

ABOUT THE AUTHOR

Andrew Sadock resides in Chicago, Los Angeles, and northeastern Michigan. During summers, he serves as owner and captain of an authentic wooden tall ship, *Red Witch*, a 77-foot, 41-ton wooden two-masted gaff-rigged schooner. During winters, Mr. Sadock serves as a holistic life coach/consultant, energyworker, qi gong instructor, motivational speaker, and performing musician; he also offers silent meditation sails—featuring whale and dolphin sightings—on the Pacific Ocean from Marina Del Rey.

Mr. Sadock has the intention to serve as a professor to introduce a curriculum of holistic philosophy/psychology/energetic medicine to universities adapted from three books he has authored that comprise the Anatomy of the Human Fabric Trilogy. Additionally, he intends to create a non-profit foundation to serve underprivileged children aboard his tall ship and sailboat (in Chicago and Los Angeles, respectively).

He practiced holistic energywork and bodywork in Chicago, San Francisco, and at Esalen Institute (Big Sur). He has written this series of three books—*Anatomy of the Human Fabric Trilogy*—on holistic philosophy/psychology/energetics. Mr. Sadock also created a screenplay adaptation of the first book he wrote, which chronicles a profound true tale of synchronicity (chronicling an inadvertent shift from medical school to a decade-long residence, meditation, and journey with shamans/indigenous healers, and the eventual practice of holistic medicine/psychology/energetics).

Mr. Sadock's background includes experience as an energyworker, certified qi gong teacher, licensed massage therapist, child advocate, musician (composer, lyricist, instrumentalist, vocalist), U.S. Merchant Marine Officer (100-ton qualification), sailor, motorcyclist, rugby player, and rugby coach.

In addition to the above three books and screenplay, Mr. Sadock has created two CDs, *Yang* (world percussive jazz) and *Yin* (contemplative ambient), designed to enhance inner vibration.

CONTACT INFORMATION

Email: Andrew@AndrewSadock.com
asadock@gmail.com
URL: AndrewSadock.com
(773) 439.0948

www.ingramcontent.com/pod-product-compliance
Lightning Source LLC
Chambersburg PA
CBHW022135080426
42734CB00006B/372